MW00997358

THE ONLY ANSWER TO CANCER

DEFEATING THE ROOT CAUSE OF ALL DISEASE

DR. LEONARD COLDWELL
INSTINCT BASED MEDICINE™

HEALING NATURE

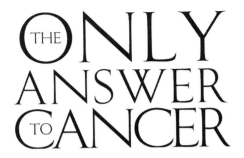

THE ONLY ANSWER TO CANCER

Copyright © 2010
Leonard Coldwell

Published by Healing Nature Press
Springfield, MO 65807

Requests for permissions should be addressed to:

Healing Nature Press

2131 W. Republic Rd., PMB 41

Springfield, MO 65807

ISBN 978-0-9824428-7-6

Cover: Keith Locke

Book Design: Lee Fredrickson

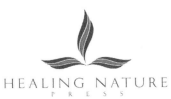

HEALING NATURE
P R E S S

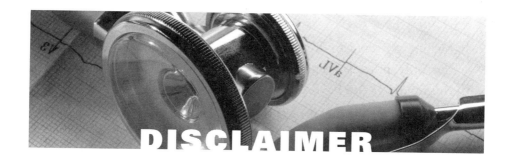

DISCLAIMER

Disclaimer: For over 20 years I have been curing cancer. I have found the one and only remedy, and it is God's/Nature's Cure. You are created to be healthy, happy and successful. You are not supposed to suffer for the financial profit of the pharmaceutical industry or medical profession or the power-and money-hungry American Cancer Society and all of their pawns in politics, the media or "self-help groups."

It is my opinion that the main goal of government agencies like the FTC or FDA (they have to legally be dissolved, and fast!), and other organizations is to protect the profits of the pharmaceutical and medical industry. We have to wake up and take charge of our own health!

They definitely do not have our best interests in mind or they would never have made laws or regulations stating that only a drug can treat, cure, diagnose or prevent any illness or condition—that is in itself absurd. No drug ever cured or prevented any disease—ever! So they knowingly set us up to suffer, pay and ultimately die.

I am telling you that the only one that can prevent or cure any disease is you! (Or God or Nature as based on your personal beliefs.)

I have personally experienced for over 30 years now that every illness can be cured, but not every patient can be cured since some people subconsciously want to die or are just not willing to do what it takes to be healthy.

Legal disclaimer: Unfortunately we live in a world of sue-happy idiots and paid destructive groups, corrupt politicians and privately owned media, so I have to legally tell you: This book and its contents do not cure, prevent, diagnose or treat any disease or condition! (Only your own self-healing powers can do that.)

The only purpose for this book is educational, for research and entertainment. If you have, or think you may have, any health condition or disease, see a competent, authorized health practitioner (if you can find one) and do not attempt any of the techniques, ideas, knowledge, suggestions or comments in this book without consulting the health professional of your choice first.

The author, the publisher and everybody involved in the creation, publication and sale of this book do not take responsibly for any outcome or result from the use of the information in this book.

Please be advised that the entire content of this book is solely the opinion of the author. Nearly everybody in the orthodox medical field disagrees with almost everything said in this book, along with the ideas, techniques and systems published herein. I, the author, don't really care! Why? Because I have the results to show, and can reproduce cancer cures anytime I want, if I would be given the legal authority to practice my IBMS™.

In my experience cancer can be cured in 2 weeks to 4 months unless too much damage has already been done by the treatment of "poison, cut and burn" of the orthodox medical profession, or if the patient is not willing or capable to do whatever it takes to experience true heath. In cases where the patient is already far too damaged by the health challenges he or she endures, the techniques may not work–but in my experience that is very rare.

So, it's up to you and your God-given rights; your right of freewill, your right to choose, your right of self-defense, and all the wonderful rights our great constitution has given us to do whatever we choose! But you have to do this at your own risk and responsibly, and accept the consequences of your decision and actions. We do not take any responsibly for anything you decide to do.

Any cure you experience is solely because of you the reader. You are the only one responsible for your own success or failures based on your actions.

And here it is, in my opinion and experience and with absolute conviction: *The Only Answer to Cancer!*

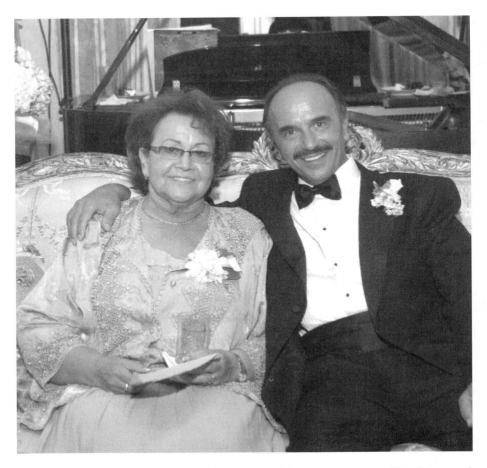

Mama Coldwell, summer 2009, was cured by her own son, Dr. Leonard Coldwell, from liver cancer, liver cirrhosis and hepatitis C in the terminal state over 35 years ago. Today, she is the healthiest and most vital and living proof of Dr. Coldwell's ability to cure cancer!

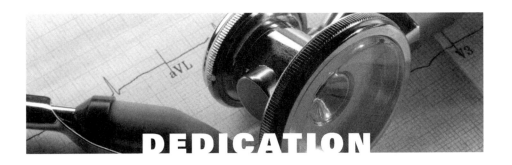

DEDICATION

This book is dedicated to the fight against cancer and all of the people who will not settle for a death sentence or a life filled with suffering just because a doctor tells them so. And to the strongest women in the world, my mother and all the wonderful people that made me, my success and my system and its publication possible:

My wonderful wife Tina for her understanding and endless support.

My perfect personal assistant, editor and friend Kelly Wallace for always being there for me.

My brother Jens for his constant support and for pushing me further when I thought I could go no further.

My great friends and supporters: Dr. Rima Laibow, Dr. Betty Martini, Dr. Thomas Hohn, Dr. Holger Crone, Prof. Dietrich Wilkening, Maj. Gen. Albert N. Stubblebine III (US Army, Ret.) Juergen Kettner, Fred Van Liew, Will Green, John Eagle Freedom, Kevin Roslansky, Lee Fredrickson, Andrew Bruex and most of all my dear and loyal friend Kevin Trudeau!

And to everybody who's supported me and my ideas along the way, as well as my former patients for their trust, my more than 2.2 million seminar attendees and over 7 million readers for their support and kind words along the way.

I thank you all!

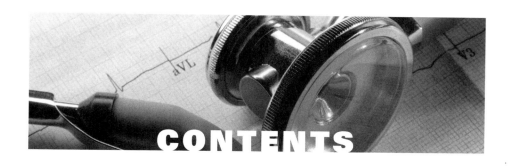

CONTENTS

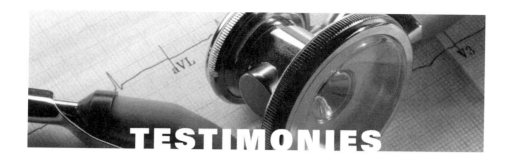

TESTIMONIES

WHAT INTERNATIONAL LEADERS ARE SAYING ABOUT THE AUTHOR

Dr. Leonard Coldwell is a remarkable asset: brilliant, brave, innovative and creative. Motivated by the devastation of cancer in his family, Dr. Coldwell set out to find the cure for cancer - and found it, curing his mother and 35,000 people found him - and came away cured of their disease. Not surprisingly, German authorities persecuted him until he was forced to close his cancer hospitals there and came to the US where he continued his ground-breaking work.

I regard Dr. Coldwell as a true treasure and I treasure both my friendship and professional relationship with him. I urge you to read this book carefully and then share it with everyone you know facing cancer themselves or in their loved ones.

Yours in health and freedom,
Rima E. Laibow, MD
Medical Director
Natural Solutions Foundation
www.GlobalHealthFreedom.org

The Only Answer to Cancer is one of those rare books which can save your life or someone else's life. Natural Cancer treatment is very dear to my heart since I was diagnosed with terminal cancer in 1994 but, through totally natural means, lost the cancer and gained optimal health through its treatment. You can, too, following the deep wisdom in this book.

The cancer establishment doesn't want you to know that you have safe, effective and inexpensive natural options since cancer is the single most profitable disease ever encountered by mankind. Brave leaders like Dr. Coldwell are dangerous to the industry that depends on your illness and your ignorance: nowhere is that more true than the multi-trillion dollar cancer industry.

Dr. Coldwell is a gifted doctor whose special gifts are curing people and telling the truth about disease—and the industry that wants to keep you as sick as possible as long as possible. His pioneering work has brought him the success and reputation to back up what he says. I believe in his new book, The Only Answer to Cancer, because I know that Dr. Coldwell's work has helped huge numbers of patients with cancer and other terminal diseases. I am proud to have Dr. Coldwell as my fellow health freedom fighter.

Yours in health and freedom,
Maj. Gen. Albert N. Stubblebine III
(US Army, Ret.)
President
Natural Solutions Foundation
www.GlobalHealthFreedom.org

"It was an honor to be able to work with Dr. Coldwell for all these years and to witness the daily miracles that seem for Dr. Coldwell just simple "normal." I have seen patients that have been on their deathbed recovering from cancer or patients with no hope. I have known Dr. Coldwell's main miracle his own mother that Dr. Coldwell cured from liver cancer in a terminal state over 3 decades ago, for many years and I have researched all of her files and data and the more I read about how sick she was with her Hepatitis C, liver cirrhoses and terminal liver cancer, and the more I read the more impressive her total healing became to me.

I have seen many patients that Dr. Coldwell cured from cancer and other diseases like Multiple Sclerosis and Lupus and Parkinson's and even muscular dystrophy and many, many more and I am still in constant awe of Dr. Coldwell's talent and results. I am so glad I could study with him personally and to learn his IBMS™ directly from him. When he left Europe, he left a huge hole, a massive empty space, in the world of cancer treatment behind. I am honored and excited about the possibilities that Dr. Coldwell opened up for me as his Master student and that he has the trust in me and my talents, that he picked me as his successor when he retired from his work with patients. "

—Dr. Thomas Hohn MD NMD Licensed IBMS Therapist™
www.goodlifefoundation.com

Research in the USA and Australia reveals the 5 year survival benefit to chemotherapy patients is 2%, that's a single week, for living in hell for 5 years! Orthodox medicine butchers, burns and poisons patient-victims and frequently shortens their lives, meanwhile their life savings are transferred to the medical establishment. Dr. Coldwell is a heroic pioneer who has delivered thousands from this fatal ordeal. This humanitarian's vital book may save you or a loved one from a world of pain. Step "out of the box" and study it carefully for your own sake.

—Dr. Betty Martini, D.Hum, Foun
Mission Possible International

My son is my hero and the hero of countless other people that he touched with his outstanding greatness. God gave him the special talent and power to heal. I was his secretary when he had his first office when he was just 14 years old and I saw so many miracles happen every single day. I always believed in my son and his abilities to help other people to overcome their life's challenges and when he simply cured them in the shortest amounts of time.

I know what it means to get a death sentence. When the doctor told me that I had liver cancer in the terminal state and only had 2 months to a maximum of 2 years to live, I locked myself in my bedroom and cried for 3 days. It was my own son that gave me the reason and motivation to fight and to live. It was my own son that cured me from a terminal disease with no hope of healing or survival 38 years ago. Now I am 74 years old and in the best shape, health and vitality of my life. I owe this to my wonderful son, Dr. Leonard Coldwell, the greatest healer of our time.

Even if he always says: "It isn't me that has cured my patients, they have cured themselves" I still know and insist that it was him and the powers God gave him that cured me and all the other patients. Without him we would not exist anymore!

Son, you gave us the strength to fight, to hang in and to survive. You gave us your love, trust, honesty, and your knowledge, but most of all your inner strength. In turn, this gave us the strength to believe in ourselves and our future. It was always you that motivated your patients, readers and seminar attendees to get up and fight and to get up and walk and to never, ever accept any other outcome but total health, success and happiness. It was, is and always will be for me: Always YOU!

Your loving Mother,
Mama Coldwell, summer 2009

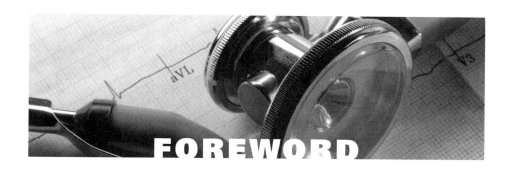

FOREWORD

Dr. Leonard Coldwell in his book *The only Answer to Cancer*, in my own experience as a professional nutritionist for over 40 years, has enabled me to fully appreciate the vast knowledge he has expressed in this book. Dr. Leonard Coldwell's comprehension grasp of the God-given remedial capabilities is very impressive. His approach enables the human body to fully express the healing nature that God has designed. Dr. Coldwell fully understands, not only the nature laws of biology that human body is governed by, but he also expresses the in depth comprehension of spirit, soul and body. Many nutritionists just focus on diet and nutrition without factoring in the emotional, physiological and spiritual aspect. Dr. Coldwell states that we are what we believe, think and eat.

I have always believed, and my clinical and personal experience has confirmed, that the human body is "Spiritually and Vibrationally induced, Electrically and Chemically empowered and biologically and genetically carried out." Recent studies and revelations in cellular biology by prominent scientists has confirmed that our spiritual beliefs and the thoughts we entertain not only help us with our fears, anxieties and the relief of stress but also upon our genetic switches and markers which enable us to have a profound effect of the status of our health. After reading Dr. Coldwell's book, I see that he has made the connection into this concept that I myself believe and follow. His concept of instinct based medicine is fully in accord to living toward natural law as created by God.

Dr. Coldwell conveys that the human body has this marvelous ability to heal itself when presented with the right circumstances in accord with its biological design. My healthy journey which has been similar to Dr. Coldwell is a recommendation that this book is a must read for anybody that wants to gain a comprehensive understanding and full appreciation beyond solely the study of nutrition.

—Fred Bisci

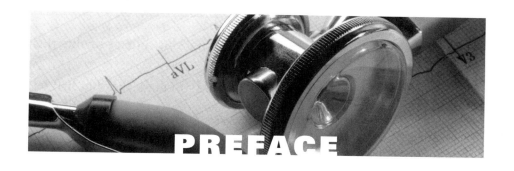

THERE ARE NO INCURABLE DISEASES ONLY INCURABLE PEOPLE

When I was seven years old, I remember my mother crying constantly from intense pain. I watched helplessly as doctors gave her painkillers and shots so that she would be more comfortable. Due to complications from gallbladder surgery performed by a medical doctor, my mother developed liver cirrhosis of the worst kind. Her liver was inflamed and she was constantly in horrible pain. When I turned 12, my mother's liver cirrhosis progressed into terminal liver cancer. The doctors gave her a maximum of two years to live. They stated that there was no hope; no one had ever recovered from this kind of advanced cancer.

The doctors suggested that she had to learn to live with the pain and make the best out of the time she had left. Imagine what this meant to a little boy like me. All I could think about was if my mother would still be alive when I got home from school that day. In fact, the first thing I would do when I got home from school was open my mother's bedroom door to see if she was still alive. I would do this every morning as well.

While she was in the hospital, I was constantly worried. I was afraid that my mother would die. I cried more during this time of my life than any other time.

My mother and I only had each other. My biological father had left us because he did not want a sick wife. It was probably best that he left because he abused my mother and made our lives miserable. We were better off without him, but we were financially really poor.

With no means of financial support, I became the sole breadwinner for our family. I cleaned restaurants before school and worked in a sandwich shop after school. It was the only way that I could put food on the table and a roof over our heads.-

I also paid for medical treatment and alternative therapies that the health insurance did not cover. We had nothing to lose. The medical profession had completely given up on my mother and refused to treat her anymore. The only things they gave her were painkillers.

Of course, my experience with the pharmaceutical and medical profession occurred in Germany. Things may have turned out differently if we were living elsewhere but there is no way to tell now. I tried desperately to find a cure for my mother's cancer. We tried everything from alternative medicine to homeopathy to healers from all over the world… nothing seemed to work.

I read every book about healing that I could get my hands on. I went to countless seminars, studied herbs, hypnotherapy, and tried all kinds of medical and alternative therapies, even new age stuff. I was desperate to help my mother and was willing to try anything. I did try it all, believe me.

I was constantly experimenting with on my mother. It was trial and error, and we had nothing to lose. Finally, our retired family doctor sat down with me to explain the functions and connections regarding medicine. She studied with me, explained medical procedures and helped me to understand the way of medical thinking and theories. While studying naturopathic medicine, I discovered that new age stuff does not work. Unfortunately, neither does modern medicine. But, if we combine our forces of natural healing and the result-producing knowledge of modern medicine we can create the perfect way to health.

Through cutting, poisoning and medical malpractice they murdered my Dad

My father passed away recently after a long battle with colon cancer. His death is a sobering reminder that conventional medicine is a miserable failure when it comes to treating chronic illness. Drugs and surgery are not the answer. It is too late for my father, but I share my experience with you so that you won't make the same mistake (My biological father, who lost his leg due to malpractice, died of stomach cancer in the same way that my "real" father died of his colon cancer treatment.)

Over the past four years, the medical establishment poisoned, burned and slaughtered my father. Doctors gave him bad advice and frightened him into surgery, which ultimately cost him his life. It grieves me deeply, because his death could have been prevented.

I've spent the past 30 years showing people how to activate their body's natural healing power. I have seen thousands of people recover from disease, but I could not save my father because he was fraudulently and purposefully misled by doctors, who preyed on his simplicity and fear.

My system could have awakened the extraordinary healing power of his body, and its natural ability to heal itself. Instead, my father trusted his doctor, and it cost him his life.

When my father was diagnosed with colon cancer, I urged him to leave Germany and come to America so that I could treat him. Colon cancer is something that I usually cure within three weeks with an almost 100% success rate. I assured my Dad that recovery would be fast and easy. I was completely convinced that I could cure him!

My Dad was a simple, hard working, honest man who wanted to be straightforward with his doctor. My Dad told his doctor that he was going to America to get cured by his son.

In response, the doctor said his tumor was so large that it would burst in the airplane. The doctor persuaded my Dad to have surgery immediately. "The surgery is simple and easy," he insisted. "The hospital does this type of surgery every day. Get the surgery first, and then fly to America."

My trusting father believed his doctor. He was convinced that the doctor was the ultimate authority, having his best interest at heart. The doctor said that he was doing me a favor. It would be easier for me to treat him if the tumor was gone. So my Dad decided to surprise me and followed his doctor's orders.

Nobody told my Dad that the tumor had grown into his spine and was impossible to remove. The doctors were fully aware of this and they still proceeded with surgery. Later, I found out that the doctors wanted to keep my Dad away from me. They were aware of my track record as a natural health practitioner. I was a threat to their way of doing business.

Death is a hard pill to swallow. Conventional medicine took the life of my unborn sister (with a use of a "new "drug while my mom was pregnant without telling my mom that they used the drug,) my grandmother, father and countless family members. Why do they trick and deceive us into destroying our mind, body and spirit? They're motivated by profit and greed. At the very least, they are incompetent and ignorant. Conventional medicine is a mega trillion-dollar industry. It employs millions of people and produces astronomical profits for hospitals and the pharmaceutical industry. Any alternative that is safe, natural and effective is a threat to the entire system. It cuts into their bottom line.

Doctors are also usually completely ignorant about nutrition, vitamins and energy. They parrot the same old stuff that they've read in medical textbooks or learned in college. For this reason, they have a limited frame of reference. Their teachings are outdated and obsolete. Most M.D.s do not have any formal education in diet and nutrition.

My Dad's tumor was at least 20 years old, but now he needed surgery immediately. He had no pain or discomfort and this tumor could have remained for years without injury.

On the operating table, the doctors cut my Dad open and disfigured him in the worst possible way. They removed the tumor, but left a large portion of it in there. After the surgery, Dad suffered from chronic pain. He developed a problem with his lungs. The doctors overlooked my Dad's methothelioma, which he developed at age 18 from working with asbestos. His condition was previously in remission (with the help of nutrition and vitamin supplements) but now it was back in the form of a respiratory infection. He nearly died and then he got pneumonia. His life was on thin ice again.

To "help" my father, the criminals in white lab coats performed emergency cervical surgery. They persuaded him to try chemotherapy, which is a poisonous form of chemical warfare that is leftover from World War I and II. Later they burned my Dad with radiation, another ineffective treatment. None of this cured or treated anything. Radiation and chemotherapy treatment is based upon the absurd hope that if you kill bad things then your cancer will disappear and your health will return. The problem is that chemo zaps and kills vital organisms and the cause of cancer is never considered. With these treatments, my father was poisoned, burned and nearly died.

Most cancer victims die from the side effects of treatment, rather than the disease itself. Of course, a death certificate will probably list heart failure as the cause of death, but the side effects are to blame.

My Dad's tumor grew more aggressively after the surgery and eventually exploded. Typically, surgery suppresses your immune system, which causes the cancer to grow even faster. That's when the doctors insist that your cancer is rapidly progressing and getting worse.

A doctor's manipulation tactics are so obvious. First, they give a devastating diagnosis, then life-or-death scare tactics to lure you into surgery. This is followed by chemo and radiation all of which will drain your wallet dry.

Doctors know that if you talk to other cancer victims and their friends and family, you'll hear plenty of horror stories: treatments gone awry with unimaginable pain and suffering. You will discover that many cancer victims have died. Ironically, what most doctors are afraid of is alternative, non-invasive healing methods that may actually cure people. That's scary, because it affects their bottom line.

Even scarier is that doctors can't identify the root cause of cancer and how to cure it. They lie to people when they insist that cancer treatments are effective. They do more harm than good. No cancer victims have been cured because of chemo and radiation. Cancer survivors have recovered in spite of their therapy. Even if you deny all treatment you have a 27% chance that your cancer will go into remission. With the help of alternative medicine, you have a 50% chance of recovery. As a natural health practitioner, I have a 92.3% cancer recovery rate with patients who had no prior medical treatment. The medical profession has a cancer recovery rate of 3%. That is significantly less than the 24% who recovered with no treatment at all.

Before his death, I was able to see my father one last time. He had countless surgeries, chemo, radiation treatments, and the doctors even created a separate exit for his bowel movements.

At that time, I realized that it was too late to help my Dad. There was not enough left of him to initiate health and healing. I tried everything I could to give him a couple of more years of pain-free living, but the side effects of the medical treatment were completely devastating.

Dad's last year was unbearable for him and the family. The medical treatment left nothing but an empty hollow of a man. Chronic pain made life unbearable and grim. After the medical establishment drained his life savings, they sent him home from the hospital, and my 70 year-old-mother was forced to take care of him around the clock. He was not even a shadow of the fierce, funny and lovable man that he once was. Now he cried constantly from pain, his body was stuffed with plastic tubes for artificial respiration and elimination. He was totally incapacitated of doing anything on his own. The doctors sent him home to die. This infuriates me! The worthless medical treatment cost him everything he had. They took his life savings as well as his livelihood. They even kept Dad from visiting me for alternative treatment and made notes of this in his medical file.

A doctor's potential to harm has been recognized since ancient times. The first written set of laws in human history, the Code of Hammurabi, was created nearly 4,000 years ago in Babylon. The Code established rewards and punishments for medical practice, and other professions. A surgeon who successfully saved a patient from a tumor received 10 shekels; one whose patient died under the knife had his hands cut off. "First, do no harm" became the main code of the medical profession.

It shouldn't be, "first, make all the money you can and then move on to the next victim." These doctors should be punished, not financially rewarded for their losses.

When conventional medicine murdered my father, I declared war on the cruel and de-humanizing way that sick people are abused, tortured, disfigured, slaughtered, poisoned, radiated and killed in the name of modern medicine. The medical agenda and motive is clear. They don't know what cures people, but they are willing to risk lives in order to make money and stay in business. This hypocrisy and double-standard includes government agencies, politicians, medical profession and, most of all, the pharmaceutical industry. It should be brought to a grinding halt. This will only happen if people have the courage to take a stand, challenge the establishment, think for themselves and claim full responsibility for their health.

Sometimes it is so much harder to help your own family and friends (as the Bible states: the prophet in his own land....) because you are too familiar and close to them. They know you as a child and as simple human being and instead tend to trust a stranger.

The struggle at the beginning

Of course I have made many mistakes in the search for my life's purpose, my true personality and my personal development. However, that was a good thing because you can learn from personal experience and your mistakes. Someone who has never been ill or has never suffered pain cannot understand and help others in a similar situation.

I consider myself someone who constantly strives for perfection in his professional and personal development. I have never stopped working at perfecting my system of self-help and self-healing and developing myself and my personal skills.

With this motivation, I read every book I could find about healing, orthodox medicine, natural healing, metaphysics and related matters, in the hope that I would find a way to heal my mother. By the age of sixteen I knew more about various healing methods than many therapists. I attended back-to-back seminars and explored every possible means to gather more information on the subject of healing. I studied natural healing, explored all available information, researched, learned and discovered!

I discovered something "new" that is actually as old as humanity itself: The only help is self-help and the only way to healing is self-healing.

It is of course difficult to say to a person, who is severely ill: "Get up and walk!" Sometimes it is almost impossible to tell a person plagued by pain: "Start to fight, find the causes that have led to your illness, take charge of your own fate, recognize your mistakes, weaknesses and errors and eliminate them. Activate the powers of your subconscious and heal yourself—now, here, today, immediately!"

I have known many people that I could not approach like that. Nonetheless, many of them gave me just enough information to allow me insight into their illnesses. For example, my grandfather returned from a prison camp in Russia, ill, maltreated, and exhausted. His liver had shrunk to a small round ball and doctors agreed that the end of his life was near. He also suffered from black lung from being a coal miner all his life. However, my grandfather began to fight back. He read books about natural nutrition and behavior regimens based on natural methods. He managed to change his attitude and took the responsibility for his life in his own hands! He reached such a high level of self-awareness that he was able to tell his subconscious: I shall not die; I shall become healthy, healthier than ever before! He used this program with admirable perseverance and discipline. My grandfather regained his health and became extremely vigorous; his mind remained active until he died at the age of 86, after the medical profession murdered him. He had to go into a hospital with some lung problems. They put him in a bathroom until a room was ready. He had a high fever and the bathroom was not heated in the middle of a very cold winter. He had no real sheet and just the hospital gown on. They forgot about him for almost 24 hours in this cold bathroom. When they finally found him, he had pneumonia and high fever and died shortly after that.

Looking at his outstanding healing process and observing similar experiences of other people, it became clear to me that there is always a way. You must just be willing to search your path, recognize it and follow it faithfully.

My Uncle Fritz also showed me that the impossible can become possible. At this time, my knowledge about the system of healing was already well developed. Uncle Fritz became my first real success. He had retired early because he could no longer lift his arms due to a chronic inflammation of his shoulder joints. I succeeded in helping him. Many of my relatives, friends and acquaintances have been cured of all kinds of health problems through my method of natural healing. These problems included migraine headaches, stomach ulcers, intestinal problems and more.

Around that time, life confronted me with a task that left me in fear and horror.

My then girlfriend was diagnosed with an advanced case of cervical cancer. I already thought of myself as a great "healer." However, I knew then that I had to improve and escalate all the information that I had learned up to that point. I was fighting illness, time and fear. After six months, however, my girlfriend was completely healed. Today, many years later, she is physically fit and full of vitality.

Steps to healing

My mother's case showed me how difficult the task of healing is and what it entails.

Despite her cancer, she opened a coffee shop with my father even though money was in short supply. My biological father had problems of his own: he had lost a leg due to medical malpractice and could stand only with the help of a wooden prosthesis. Sometimes he bled; sometimes he cried from excruciating pain. Managing the coffee shop required that both of my parents spend a lot of time on their feet. They opened the coffee shop because they hoped to earn enough money for the pursuit of alternative methods of healing that their health insurance would not cover. Indeed, my mother went to see many doctors, chiropractors, miracle healers and quacks in Germany, Holland, Switzerland

and Austria. Anyone who has been in a similar situation understands what I am talking about. What happened? Nothing! But I did notice that my mother's energy level increased slowly. I witnessed how her confidence and strength steadily increased. Together, we discovered that the botched gallbladder operation was the cause of the horrible suffering she endured for so many years. A second operation revealed that only half of the gallbladder had been removed and that a new stone was lodged in the remaining portion of the gallbladder, blocking the passageways and poisoning the liver. Consequently everything in that part of her body was poisoned and destroyed.

A new phase in my life and work

My mother and I began to practice the method that led to my current **Instinct Based Medicine™ System** with an iron will, self-discipline and faith. The miracle healing of my mother took place. Even my sister developed cancer over 28 years ago but is in perfect health today.

I hope that you too will experience such a miracle, if you are suffering in a similar manner. We all deserve to be healthy and live without pain. You too are probably a mother, father, brother, or sister to someone and your family is concerned about you and shares your pain.

I am telling you all this, because these events led to the next step in my research. I came to the conclusion that self-pity is a destructive force from within that can destroy people. Only the sick person can cure himself. If you want to help a patient you must motivate him, because he alone can facilitate the healing in his body, soul, and spirit. Indeed, only the individual's own will, spirit and motivation can set the necessary healing process in motion.

There are, of course, many outstanding therapists, whose accomplishments deserve unlimited recognition. When you are ill, consult a doctor immediately but don't trust only one opinion, ask a lot of questions and most of all make your own educated decisions. It is your health and your life. Don't trust it in the hands of others! However, the doctor should not be viewed as a healer, but rather as a partner in a joint effort to bring the afflicted individual's body and soul, which are out of sync, back into a state of natural balance. Even the best doctors can only prescribe a therapy or medication which might help to suppress the symptoms, but they cannot and will not heal you. The healing process lies within the individual's body, his immune system and his self-healing power. Remember that the medical profession is like any other trade, there are always more incompetent people than competent ones.

By now you should understand that idleness, crying and self-pity will not make you healthy. Education and self-help is the only way.

My personal quest for healing

I know what I am talking about because I have gone through it myself. For many years I lived with continuous pain and illness. Doctors and physicians could not help me even with surgery. I had chronic bronchitis, severe eye problems, chronic spine problems, gallstones, colic, liver problems and a two year infection that affected almost all the organs in my body. I invested more than 1.6 million dollars into my teeth and had close to 4,000 hours in the dentist chair with no satisfying solution until today. The pain and suffering I experienced made me wish for my own death. I am telling you this so that you won't think: yes, it is easy to talk. I speak from personal experience. I have not only had serious medical problems, I have studied and practiced health. They wanted to take my appendix out because they did not correctly diagnosis my gallbladder problem. That was the start of the invention of the **Instinct Based Medicine™ System.**

I started my quest to find the answer to cancer and other diseases by studying every successful healing technique worldwide, and I learned about all the alternative or natural forms of healing available. I discovered why people got cancer and how they got healthy after they had it, and why others just died. And so I became one of the leading experts for cancer in Europe long before I graduated from medical/naturopathic medical school.

I then specialized as a general physician in cancer with a particular emphasis on cancer patients who had been deemed incurable by their physicians. Working with these people, I learned that there is always hope, there is always a way, and there will always be patients that will regain their health, no matter what the diagnosis or obstacles. Most importantly, I learned that I was not the healer, I was only the conduit for my patient to pass on the knowledge and tools and training he or she needed to reactivate the immune system and stimulate self-healing powers so that the patient could achieve optimum health.

The bottom line, and the most important lesson I learned from working with over 35,000 patients with so-called incurable diseases, is that nobody can cure anybody; only the sick can cure themselves. (Many of you know that I am Mega Best Selling Author and Consumer Advocate Kevin Trudeau's personal physician as well as the consultant to many of the rich and famous and the many of the world's leading companies. I do not work with patients anymore because my goal is to teach and educate and to fight for Health Freedom and Patient Rights amended to the US Constitution.)

We are not failures because we are sick, unfit, or overweight. We just learned to use the powers of our brains, bodies, and immune systems in the wrong way. All too often, we are brainwashed by the media or misled by people to believe or do the wrong thing. But the good news is that there is always hope. From now on, you just need to act smarter. Make the decision to take charge of your life, happiness, and health right now! Make the commitment to live up to your potential and create the health you deserve.

93% success rate with cancer
The Bad Nenndorf Institute for Medical Statistics concluded and published:" Our research shows that Dr. Leonard Coldwell worked with over 35,000 patients with cancer and other terminal diseases and it is our conclusion that he has the highest cancer cure rate, of all researched therapists, in the World—His success rate with cancer patients, that had no orthodox medical treatment before using Dr. Coldwell's system, is 92.3% "The Berlin Health Institute conducted a two clinical studies and came to a similar conclusion in the effectiveness of the Instinct Based Medicine® System. There conclusion was also that: NPL, Hypnotism,

Meditation one other techniques do not have even 10% of the effectiveness of Dr. Leonard Coldwell's Instinct Based Medicine® System is to purposes of easier reading from now on called in this book: IBMS™ Stress Reduction System. Our studies concluded that the 20 minute IBMS™ stress reduction sessions equal the relaxation, regeneration and healing of a deep restful sleep of 7 to 8 hours.

Remember there is no magic pill, no magic healer, not secret treatment, herb or supplements that can cure you—but there is a much greater magic within each and every one of us: The love, energy and strength—the unlimited power of healing and life itself: There is the power of Nature the power of God the creates miracles every single second of our life's. We just need to be willing to acknowledge and use or even better let it work for us in our own body and the entirety of our own life!

With the deepest understanding, love, hope and the believe that you can be Happy, Healthy and Successful.

Your new friend
—Dr. Leonard Coldwell

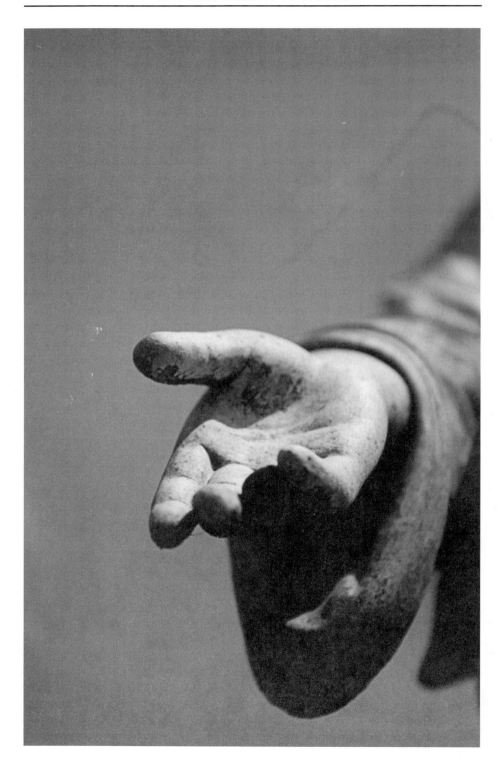

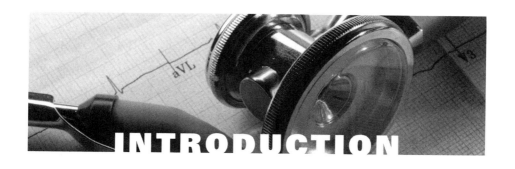

THE INSTINCT BASED MEDICINE™ SYSTEM

All illness comes from lack of energy, and the greatest energy drainer is mental and emotional stress, which I believe to be the root cause of all illness. Stress is one of the major elements that can erode energy to such a large and permanent extent that the immune system loses all possibility of functioning at an optimum level. Fact is that 86% of all illness and doctor visits are stress related and then I just learned that the Stanford University concluded after a major study that 95% of all illness is stress related. I am referring to the mental and emotional stress that is caused by continuous and/or long-term compromises against yourself. These vary from person to person, but some examples include living in unbearable relationships and marriages, doing jobs you hate or hating your boss, or experiencing problems with family, all of which lead to you compromising your sense of self. Emotional and mental stress comes from living with feelings of constant fear, doubt, hopelessness, lack of self-esteem, worry, and, most of all, always compromising your inner feelings, instincts, and personal needs. The main component of all these energy drainers is fear. But the Bible tells us over 100 times: Not to fear and to trust in God! Your faith can heal you from fear!

The solution is to start by defining what it is in your life that keeps you from feeling happy. Can you answer the question of why you don't respect yourself enough? Or love yourself? Now identify what needs to change or happen in your life to make you feel good about yourself and your personal environment. What is it that you don't want to do, accept, or take anymore from yourself, your spouse, your children, your boss, or your coworkers? Is there someone in your life that makes you feel badly that needs to go? What are your wildest dreams and goals? Looking at your life, what is it that always takes away your energy, and where do you compromise your personal needs and feelings? Identify everything in your life that keeps you from being your true self, and start working on the development of the true you! This is the first and most important step toward achieving optimum health and happiness. And remember that happiness and hope are the most powerful healers and energy creators in your life. Pay attention to your instincts, listen to your inner voice, and start loving and respecting yourself so that you behave according to your true personality. You need to accept the statistical fact that the medical doctor or medical profession is the number one cause of death in America. That means you cannot rely solely on another person, the MD, with your health and life. What is even worse, is that I believe today that the US Government or better the different agencies of the Government like the FDA and FTC are the leading cause of death in this world because of their manipulations, suppressions, rules and regulations that prevent natural health, natural healing methods, natural cures, healing foods and supplementation and natural healers to do God's work.

If you do not live your life according to your needs, you will get or stay stressed, which will reduce your energy and eventually produce an illness. You are the only one who can change your life and improve your health. So start today by defining, creating, and living your life the way you believe is right and good for you. Create your own self-healing system—This book is my personal one for educational purposes only.

Please read the entire book first before you attempt to apply any changes for your life and health and before you do anything ask a qualified professional for help and support. You can also write to me and or licensed and practicing MD's that I have personally trained in my system (Instinct Based Medicine® - IBMS™)

A Very Clear and Short Introduction

I promised God when I sat on my mother's bed as she was screaming from pain, begging God to let her die, that if He would help me to cure her I would do everything in my power to help prevent other mothers, fathers, and their children from having to go through the same thing.

With this book I am fulfilling my promise to God and nothing will stop me. I have been threatened, shot at, my car has been bombed, they've tried to bribe me and pay me off. My books have been banned and taken off the shelves, my newspaper columns were stopped under pressure of the pharmaceutical industry. In fact, groups have been financed to defame and attack me, and so much more.

I know it will get even worse with the publication of this book because in it I tell you how easy it can be to cure cancer and how I did it. I share with you my personal experiences and opinions, and I know that anyone else can be cured of cancer as well. I have the results to prove this is true, and even my own mother was cured from Hepatitis C, liver cirrhosis and terminal liver cancer over 30 years ago. This book is a testament to God's truth and healing power, and my loving gift to you!

Be prepared because once this second book hits the mass market they will attack me personally, but they cannot attack or disprove my message and my cure—God's cure and Nature's cure. I know how to cure cancer and I will tell you how it works!

However, the pharmaceutical companies, medical industry and their pawns—like the politicians they bought off, or the criminal organizations like the FTC or FDA, or the even more harmful American Cancer society—will attack me. They will attack my character, bring up lies and create fraudulent "facts," but I really don't care. Here it is, my friend. *The only Answer to Cancer!*

Remember: **"It is only my opinion—but I may be right™"**

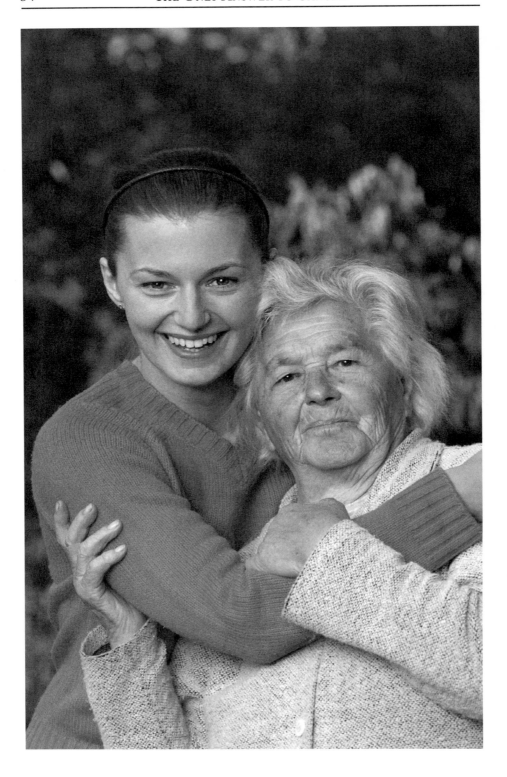

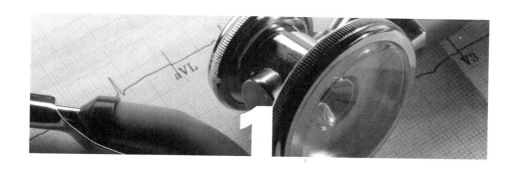

CANCER DEFINITIONS

According to our current medical model, cancer is a general term that describes a group of 100 unique diseases that are characterized by uncontrolled growth and spread of abnormal cells. But basically, cancer is cancer. They just name it based on the location where the symptoms occur, how it behaves, or how it is diagnosed and categorized in the laboratory.

If the body is designed to survive and not to destroy itself, why then would it suddenly allow the growth of extra cell tissue and kill itself? The main obstacle to finding real cures for cancer is that modern cancer treatment is rooted in the false assumption that the body sometimes tries to destroy itself. Well, it does not!

While illness appears to be something destructive and harmful for the body, it is actually an attempt by the body to cleanse and heal itself, or at least to prolong its life. For example, when you sweat, have a fever, throw up or get diarrhea when you have a cold or the flu, it is the body's way of getting rid of the toxins and microbes so it can cure itself.

Cancer cells are not part of a malicious attack on healthy cells and the body. If you have salmonella infection or poisoning, the vomiting and diarrhea are the body's way of ridding itself of the poison. If you stop the extraction of the poison you would die of the toxins. The body is smart and has learned how to survive over many generations. It does not need to be cut, poisoned or burned when it is already working on the cure!

The drastic reduction or shutdown of vital nutrient supplies to the cells of an organ is not primarily a *consequence* of a cancerous tumor, but is actually its biggest *cause*. Therefore, healthy nutrition and sufficient hydration, as well as effective breathing, are major parts for the prevention and treatment of the physical causes of cancer symptoms.

Cancer cells are normal, healthy cells that have mutated genetically so that they can live in an environment where oxygen is not available. When cells are deprived of vital oxygen (their primary source of energy), some of them will die, but others will manage to alter their genetic software program and mutate in a most ingenious way so that they can live without oxygen.

Since Nobel Prize winner Otto Warburg has scientifically proven that cancer cells cannot grow or exist in an oxygen rich environment or an alkaline environment as proved by Nobel Prize winner Max Plank, it is very simple and easy to understand that by creating an oxygen-rich and slightly alkaline body environment, the cancer cells have to disappear!

Current statistical information shows that treating cancer with suppressive methods such as radiation, chemotherapy, and surgery reduces the chance of complete remission to seven percent or less. And that is just talking about remission and the five year survival rate, not what I am talking about which is true healing and a normal life expectancy of a healthy person.

This is similar to when infections are "prevented" or suppressed through medical intervention and the liver and kidneys become less efficient in keeping the body's cell tissues free of harmful toxins, as well as the immune, lymphatic and digestive systems.

Cancer cells are normal, oxygen-dependent cells that have been genetically reprogrammed to survive in an oxygen-deprived environment. To treat cancer as if it were an illness without removing its underlying cause is nothing but malpractice.

A lack of oxygen causes a healthy cell to abandon its original genetic design and stop using oxygen. Cancer cells do not cause, but prevent death, at least for a while, until the wasting away of an organ leads to the demise of the entire organism.

A tumor is often highly toxic on the inside as it accumulates all the toxins in your body so that the poisons cannot spread into the entire body and kill you. That is the reason why biopsies and surgery— anything that cuts, opens, or hurts the protective shell of the tumor— usually leads to a very fast death. When that happens they just call it a fast growing or fast spreading form of cancer. Not that *they* spread the toxins into the patient's body and that's what killed the patient. If the causes for the cancer are properly taken care of, such an outcome can be completely avoided.

Common Answers about Cancer

If you ask around you will find that the common answers about what causes cancer are: diet, environmental, genetics, lifestyle and so on. Obviously, no one has the true answer or there would not be any cancer to begin with. But, over the years I have indeed found the root cause of all cancers and that's what I'm sharing with you in this book. Some people are very skeptical since they can't believe it's "this easy." After all, how can anything this easy be right?

Say the word "cancer" to yourself. How does it make you feel? Terrified, right? Of course! That's what the medical and pharmaceutical professions want you to feel. If you're scared to death and are even thinking about going the chemotherapy and radiation route then guess what? They've done their job and you're going to keep making them rich! They operate solely on the fear factor.

Deadly Misconceptions about Cancer

I'm here to set things straight. As I mentioned before, cancer is simply lack of energy, a lack of energy that's caused mainly by mental and emotional stress. Yes, there's a small 14% that's caused by other factors such as various toxins and so on, but if you lead a healthy lifestyle and find out the root cause of how and why you developed cancer in the first place, you don't have to worry about the "C word" anymore.

The cancer treatments forced upon us by the pharmaceutical and medical industry as they use the media to brainwash us into submission has nothing to do with prevention or cures. The early detection methods are more dangerous and cancer-causing than most people would ever believe. This is simply a way to recruit new customers. The treatments of cut, poison and burn do more harm than good and today people usually do not die of cancer anymore, they die from the effects of the treatment.

Burning or poisoning or cutting out the tumor does not cure the cancer. Cancer is a total body, mind and spirit thing. Your body develops these mutated cells and they begin to accumulate usually because of chronic mental and emotional stress.

When the MDs create scars due to radiation and surgery, this just allows new places for cancer cells to grow. Chemotherapy—a deadly poison left over from the First and Second World Wars was used to kill solders on the battlefield—causes cancer. Radiation causes cancer as well. Surgery usually makes the cancer become more aggressive and may cause it to spread through the entire body.

After they've made the cancer more aggressive they simply call it a fast-growing cancer. Instead of admitting that what they're doing doesn't work and, in fact, makes the cancer worse, they usually just shake their heads and tell the family that they caught it too late.

Cancer is cancer! It's all the same. There are no different types. Some just behave differently because of the individual circumstances of the patient or the different organ or body part they find it in. The bottom line is, don't let them scare you with complicated big words and trick you into fast surgery and deadly treatments before you get the chance to educate yourself and can make a well-informed decision.

They say you don't have time? There is always enough time! You don't have to hurry and the baloney they hand you—that you have only 3 to 6 month to live if you don't opt for their homicidal procedures—is absurd. The first thing you should do is ask them this: *"How long will I live if I go through with your treatments? I want a written guarantee."* If you do this the doctors in the white coats will back off faster than you can blink. The problem is they can always get away with these lies because after the patient dies no one is there to blame the doctors or prosecute them for their lies!

Cancer takes years to grow! So why the big hurry to start in on the painful treatments?

The reason is this, they want your money and they don't want you to have time to think about it, get educated and wiggle your way out of their greedy claws. If you get diagnosed with cancer there is always enough time to get educated and to think about it before you make any decision.

Proof Positive That Natural Cures Work

In my clinics in Europe we often used Oxygen Multi-step Therapy after Prof. Manfred von Ardenne. I have seen via camera or ultrasound how colon tumors disappear in front of our eyes when we blow ionized oxygen directly on the tumor. The founder of this therapy has published thousands of these successes.

Dr. Gerson has proven in countless cases that cancer growth stops instantly within 14 days of a fully organic raw food diet.

Dr. Batmanghelidj author of *The Body's Many Cries for Water*, has seen similar results of the body's self healing powers just by water application.

I have also seen spontaneous healings of cancerous tumors after the patient made the decision to get divorced from a spouse that was the root cause of their cancer development, or quit a job that was literally killing them.

So first, take your time. Read this book and my other book *Instinct Based Medicine How to Survive Your Illness and Your Doctor*. Read Carl

Simonton's and Bernie Siegel's books and everything you feel is right for you before you make any decision. This is your body and your life! Nobody should make decisions for you. But you must make an educated decision. Use common sense and, most of all, your instincts.

With the standard medical treatments it's often a race between which will kill you first—the treatment or the cancer!

We've talked about this before, that the average cancer cure rate of the medical "professionals" is a measly 2% - 3%. Well, what if your defense lawyer told you that you have a 97% - 98% chance of getting the death penalty? You'd want to change lawyers! Now, what if your doctor told you that you only have only 3 to 6 month to lives? Shouldn't you change doctors?

Dr. Bernie Siegel stated in one of his lectures that patients who like their doctor are more likely to die within the time frame that their doctor told them they would die in, just because on a subconscious level they don't want to prove their doctor wrong! Plus, it's the law of expectation. If you expect to die in a certain time frame you probably will.

It's a proven fact that your immune system will go down as soon as you're diagnosed with cancer because of all the negative information you've received from the media, or from seeing someone you love or know dying the horrible death of cancer. It's been ingrained into your belief system that if you have cancer you have to die. That's absolutely not true!

I have to say that I am always stunned by the fact that so many cancer patients never get rid of their individual root cause of their cancer. The past trauma, the bad relationship, the unbearable job or whatever is killing them. The second they have no pain or symptoms and they are no longer afraid of dying, they go back to the situation or behavior that made the sick in the first place and they ultimately die!

So be warned, if you don't get rid of the situations and people who are causing you stress and giving you cancer, then you're in trouble. If you don't, and even if you do "get rid of the cancer" it will always come back and usually twice as strong and fast as before, often with no cure.

Been Diagnosed With Cancer? Don't Worry, You Don't Have To Die!

In my experience, the main fear of cancer patients is not actually about the suffering and dying. What they fear most is being abandoned by their family members or their doctor. I promise you my dear new friend, *I will not abandon you!* I will fight for you and with you, and, if it comes down to it, I will help you fight against yourself!

I want to help you overcome any health challenges you may have so that you can experience the happiness and quality of life you desire and deserve. I'm convinced you don't have to suffer or die of cancer. The cure is in your own hands and this is a very empowering message to you!

However, if you're under the delusion that anybody in the medical field or pharmaceutical world is interested in a fast, safe treatment and cure for you—you will be very disappointed!

What I've discovered through the years is that cancer is the easiest condition to cure! In fact, there are over 300 proven ways to cure cancer naturally. You can eliminate tumors and mutated cell growth with:

- Vitamin B17
- 35% food grade hydrogen peroxide
- Vitamin C or Aloe Vera injections
- Essiac tea or capsules
- Turmeric
- Various mushrooms
- Oxygen or ozone therapy
- Vitamin D or sunlight
- Raw food or macrobiotic diets
- Full body and organ cleanses
- DMSO and Cesium chloride therapy
- Chinese Happy Tree
- Graviola fruit

- Triphala (Ayurvedic)
- Gerson therapy–a mixture of diet and supplementation
- Hemp or Hoxsey Therapy
- Enzyme therapy
- Hydrosol Silver
- Omega 3 fatty acids
- Eggplant (BEC–5)
- Baking soda and maple syrup
- Chelation therapy
- Photoluminescence
- Brussels sprouts, broccoli sprouts, garlic, green tea, spinach, or tomatoes
- Echinacea
- Folic acid
- Lacto-Terrine enzymes
- Saw palmetto
- Selenium
- Minerals
- Many other herbs, foods and supplements can cure the symptoms of what they call cancer.

It's true that there are many natural and easy methods of combating the symptoms of cancer, but the fact remains that 86% of all illnesses and doctor visits are stress related. This means that all of these physical treatments just mentioned can only work on 14% of the rest. This is why I have, in the opinion of many experts and institutions, the highest cancer cure rate—92.3% as concluded by the Berlin Health Institute and the Bad Nenndorf Institute for Medical statistics. Others don't even come close to this.

Most of the time I've worked only with terminal cancer patients, and I still have the highest cancer cure rate known today. The difference is that I don't treat cancer or tumors or mutated cells, I don't even treat the cancer victim. I have just learned in over 30 years of research and success how to help people to identify the root cause of their health challenges or health breakdowns and teach, coach and consult them in how to eliminate the root cause of their personal cancer—or any other disease.

The great cancer healer Dr. Simoncini M.D. in Rome has cured cancer for decades with sodium bicarbonate. He states that the medical profession has a cancer cure rate of only 2% - 3% with their mandatory orthodox therapy of chemotherapy, radiation and surgery. That means the medical profession kills nearly every patient that falls into their hands! Why? Because we know today that people don't usually die of cancer; they die from the side-effects of the treatment.

The medical profession states far different survival statistics, but this is because they manipulate studies and results. If a cancer patient is still alive five years after they've first been diagnosed, they are considered "cured"—even if they die one day or one hour later, and even if they have suffered horribly from the effects of the "cut, burn and poison" therapy.

Cancer Is a Lack of Energy

In spite of popular opinion, cancer is not a physical disease. Cancer is a mental and emotional disease caused by a lack of energy on the life energetic level. That is the reason why, even if all of the cancer treatments worked, the cancer would eventually reoccur and would be much more vicious than before.

Some think that with raw food, perfect hydration and some supplements or herbs their cancer can be cured. Absolutely not! The symptoms, the tumor, or the cell damage may disappear for awhile but it will come back unless the patient has defined and eliminated the root cause of their disease. Only then can a patient be called healthy or cured!

My Personal Quest to Cure Cancer

My first patient was my own mother. She was diagnosed with liver cancer in a terminal state over 30 years ago with a maximum prognosis of 6 month to 2 years to live. How did she develop cancer? This is how it happened: My mother nearly died from gall bladder surgery that went wrong. Because of that they gave her huge amounts of blood which in turn gave her Hepatitis C. The hepatitis turned into liver cirrhosis and later liver cancer.

The horror of those years will haunt me for the rest of my life. Often I wake up and can still hear her screaming from this unbearable pain. But to make a long story short, I cured her and she is still alive and 100% healthy for over 30 years now. My mother is 74 years old and the most vital, energetic and positive person you could ever meet.

After all seven siblings of my mom developed cancer, then my grandmother, my father and even my step-father dying of cancer, I can honestly say that I know more about cancer and its effects on a person, their family members and friends, than anybody in this world will ever know. Also, my sister had cervical cancer that I cured her from, and my first long-time girlfriend had ovarian cancer that I cured too—and this was before I ever saw a medical school from the inside.

I learned, through instinct and common sense, the way to cure cancer. Over the past decades I've perfected this system which I will share with you in these pages.

This Is Not Rocket Science!

Some may think that this is a pretty lofty claim, to say that I myself invented the cure for cancer and every other so-called incurable disease. Why is it so hard to believe? The medical profession makes cancer seem very mysterious and elusive, but the truth is, I figured the cure out all by myself. Once you finish reading *The Only Answer to Cancer*, you will also see that it's not rocket science!

So how did I actually come up with the cure? As a young man I read a lot and went to every seminar and educational workshop that they let me in to, but all of this really didn't help much. What did help was speaking to patients that had been sick and then fully recovered without the "help" of modern medicine. I was on a mission to find out how they did it. I also learned from all types of healers, finding out what worked and what didn't and then tried them on my mom since we had nothing to lose anyway. We kept what worked and left the rest.

As the years went by, I was able to cure most cancer patients in days or at least in two to six weeks—as long as the patient had not been damaged before by the murderous "therapies" of the medical profession. The only patients I ever lost during the last five years in my clinical work were patients that were destroyed by the poisons of chemotherapy, the destructive burn of radiation therapy, and/or the absurdity of surgery.

So, if you don't see references to other books or studies (with some rare exceptions) then please understand that I already knew, practiced and published all of these things 30 years ago. I had long-since been practicing what others in the world have just come out with as "brand new discoveries invented by them."

It's true! I published books 30 years ago where you can find all of the information that many say has just been discovered. Even the entire contents of the book and movie *The Secret* was published in my book: *The Unlimited Power of the Subconscious Mind* over 20 years ago. This includes the power of attraction and everything else that is suddenly a brand new discovery. In fact, the leading medical doctor in Europe, Dr. Thomas Hohn MD NMD stated: "Dr. Coldwell is so far ahead of the medical and alternative medicine world that it is like we are in kindergarten and he has graduated from University for the fourth time."

As you read this book, keep in mind that I do have, in the opinion of many leaders in the health field, the world's highest cancer cure rate. I have proven myself and my successful system over many decades because *my* cancer patients are still alive.

Where are the patients of the ones that talk the scientific talk with clinical studies and massive amounts of references? It may sound like I am bragging or have a big ego, but I just want to get this out of the way so I can finally tell you how I cure cancer and how I believe everybody else can cure him or herself of cancer—usually within weeks.

You Must Take Responsibility

My goal with this book is not to convince you of anything other than the fact that if you take responsibility for your own life, health, decisions and actions, you *can* heal. Yes, you have the God-given or Nature-given power to heal yourself, as long as you are willing to do whatever it takes to achieve this goal.

You also have to promise me that you want to live! You also have to stop feeling angry and feeling sorry for yourself. Start taking charge of your life and your actions! In order to heal, you have to be willing to change your life in all areas as necessary.

There will be no compromises, no negotiations, and no sympathy from my side, just understanding, lots of love for my fellow human being, and the will to do everything in my power to help you overcome every health challenge you may have now or in the future.

A Wakeup Call

- Stop running for the Cure!
- Stop donating money to the American Cancer Society.
- Stop wasting time with charities that raise money for cancer research.

It is all a hoax. There are already at least 300 known and proven cancer cures out there in the world. These cancer charities and research groups are simply a money-making scam. They suck the life out of you and make sure you die in about five years, not from cancer, but from the symptoms of the treatment. Cancer is the easiest body malfunction to normalize in a very short amount of time.

Stop giving yourself cancer by using the medical profession's useless and dangerous and cancer-causing early detection and diagnostic techniques. All of this is only in place to create customers for the medical community. There is no scientific proof that a mammography or other dangerous early detection methods have ever prevented anybody from getting cancer or from dying of it!

Stop putting the responsibility for your health into the hands of someone else, and most of all stop putting it into the hands of the medical profession. The medical doctor is the number one cause of death in America, and over the counter and prescription drugs are the main cause of the development of illnesses.

The medical profession has a cancer cure rate of two to three percent—What a joke! The suicide rate for medical doctors is the highest in any profession and their average lifespan of 56 years is the shortest of all professions. So why in the world would you put your life and health into their hands? Medicine is not science because it does not work as a science, it works as a religion. Simply by believing a hypothesis and not facts and science, they treat their patients. The truth is they only make money if you are sick!

Stop running from the responsibility of your own life and health. You are the only one that can make yourself sick and you are the only one that can cure yourself.

Stop feeling sorry for yourself and start living! Start healing yourself and accept the fact that you are the only one who, through decisions and actions, can determine your health, life and future on a daily basis.

There is no healing force outside the human body. If you want to be healthy and stay healthy—do something about it!

Stop believing that others have the cure for cancer and then tell me it's food, juicing, a supplement or herb—this simply isn't true! Yes, these are helpful and I recommend them, but they are not cures.

Why do you think so many people take some herbs or change their diet and get better for awhile, but later still die of cancer? *Because cancer is an energetic illness.* Cancer is in the entire existence of a person and not just in the body, and the root cause of this disease is mental and emotional stress. Yes, the root cause of all cancer is this destructive lack of energy. If you don't get rid of the root cause you cannot get rid of the cancer!

All illnesses are caused by a direct violation of God or Nature's laws. It is a violation of the use of power and freewill that you have. It is an imbalanced energy system that causes your immune system to fail. It is self-neglect, self-denial, self-hatred or subconscious suicide that leads to cancer. It's you!

It's Up To You

Whether you want to believe it or not, you gave yourself this health challenge and you can reverse it anytime you want to. But first, you must be willing to take responsibility and stop hiding behind self-pity, ignorance, arrogance or fear. This may sound harsh, but I want you to understand that you no longer have to be a victim of the medical community or your own self-destructive decisions. You are stronger than that, you are wiser!

Now it's your time to live! It is your life! You live in the here and now, and in the here and now you can choose to be happy, healthy and successful. You don't have any time to waste because your life is happening right now. Stand up and fight! Stop giving strangers complete power over your life and health.

Helplessness and hopelessness are two emotions that create cancer. If you put yourself into the hands of the medical profession what do you think you'll get more off? Yes, helplessness, hopelessness, fear and a lot of suffering!

Let me repeat:

> All cancer can be cured! Stand up and fight for yourself, your spouse, children, and all the people you love and who love you! Consider this a war book on how to fight and win against corruption, ignorance and arrogance. A way to battle against fear, loneliness, false information, manipulation, and most of all the media (that false prophet!) along with the medical profession and pharmaceutical industry, and anyone else who makes money on your pain, suffering and ultimate death. Give them the finger and start fighting back! It is your right!
>
> *Like Jesus said, "Stand up and walk!"*

Don't Treat the Cancer Treat the Person!

Just listen to how the medical doctors talk: "We treat the tumor, we kill the cancer cells, we fight the cancer, and we treat the cancer." To do this is like fighting against a riptide. No matter how much you fight, you'll still be pulled under the water!

Cancer is just the symptom of a life that lacks energy. To cure cancer, all they would have to do is help the patient to define the root cause of his or her individual illness and teach them how to eliminate this cause. Once this is accomplished, what they call cancer will disappear on its own.

But here's the catch: There is no money in you getting healthy, so nobody in the medical profession is interested in giving you advice on how to stay healthy or get healthy in the most natural way possible. Plus, no one has ever trained these medical doctors in natural healing techniques, healing diets, supplementation and herbs for effective stress reduction. In my experience, stress is always the cause of every illness!

It's important to understand our nature and not to separate the health challenge, the illness, or the cancer from the person. Cancer is not a separate living being that can be fought without harming the person that the cancer is a part of.

Cancer is nothing but mutated and deformed half-dead cells that multiply themselves in that area of your body. Cancer is nothing new to the body, it's simply a problem of free radicals which are always present in the body from the day we are born, but our immune system usually gets rid of them all the time from your first day of life onward. Statistically, we all get cancer at least six times in our life and if no one tells us about it (such as in the early detection fraud) it usually goes away the same way it developed in the first place: It simply undevelops itself!

If you have the bad luck of getting your yearly physical and have been tricked into going to cancer screenings or early detection procedures, and at the same time you just happen to have some cancer buildup in your body, the medical professional will scare you instantly into surgery, chemo and radiation. They always use fear as their weapon against you!

By the way, if they kill someone too fast or too obviously with their barbaric medieval treatments they just say, "We caught it too late. If we would have gotten it earlier we could have saved him."

All of this is a huge lie; they cannot cure anybody with poisoning, cutting and burning! Did you know that breast cancer, for example, grows about 7 to 10 years in a woman's breast before they can even find and diagnose it? Once they do, it's supposedly a matter of days or even hours that the poor woman has to get her breast cut off or maimed. The cancer grows in there for nearly a decade but to avoid having you think about alternative treatments and possibly skipping out on their income generating scheme, they scare you into instant surgery or treatment. After they cut you open and bombard your with their poisons and burn you with radiation you are much too weak to escape their claws and they will usually end up "treating you to death."

Cancer is Cancer

To make it look like the MDs know what they're talking about and what they're doing they give cancer different names based on Latin or Greek or Spanish languages to try to impress you and give the illusion that they know what it is and how to get rid of it, but they don't.

Cancer is cancer, there aren't different types. They just name it after the place in the body where it is and how it behaves. That's it! Let me repeat, cancer is cancer, it's all the same! Even if the medical community comes up with more complicated words and names based on the difference in structure or based on specific tests, it's still the same cancer.

Have you noticed that they always make up names for illnesses? Your doctor won't be happy until he finds a label to put on your disease. I don't even believe there is some illness called "cancer." These are just specific symptoms, and when they occur they just call it cancer and create the illusion—or delusion—that it is something separate from you. Something that is alive and existing on its own within your body and it needs to be cut out, burned out or poisoned to death. But since these tumors or cell mutations are a part of your own body, if they kill them they kill you too!

For example, they call a specific condition related to bones that have holes in them and are brittle, osteoporosis. Osteoporosis is simply Latin for bones with holes in them. So, to say that osteoporosis causes bones with holes in them is like saying, bones with holes in them cause bones with holes in them! How ridiculous is that?

It is all just a big hoax and they speak Latin so you don't understand what they're saying, and to let you know that they have no idea what you have, where it comes from and how to treat it naturally without any side effects. Plus, if they use exotic words it usually impresses the patient who now believes that since their doctor knows what condition they have they also know how to cure it. Wrong!

These so-called medical professionals are not even trained to cure anyone, nor have they studied health. They've studied pathology, illness, death and chemical intervention to suppress the symptoms in hopes that in the meantime your own body cures itself on its own. If you do heal, they know that you'll believe the doctor or their drug did the healing. But today it's even worse because they unknowingly or intentionally give you new diseases, symptoms and conditions so that they have something new to treat all the time.

Let's face it, a doctor's office is a business, just like your deli, butcher shop or bakery, and if all of their patients were healthy they would have no income and would soon go bankrupt. To avoid going broke, they make sure to constantly create new business for themselves.

The newest money making trick is all of these diagnostic gimmicks and early detection scams they use to make money even on healthy people, but this also creates new customers. They *always* find something to treat you for or they just make it up, much like the cholesterol lie. You die of not enough cholesterol, not because of too much. There has never been a fatal heart attack caused by cholesterol ever, they are caused by acidosis and a chemical reaction, and not by cholesterol. And, the cholesterol drugs themselves cause cancer, hardening of the liver, and all kind of cardiovascular diseases, but, this is for another book.

Cancer Is the Easiest Malfunction to Reverse

Cancer is not the big myth you've been lead believe. Cancer is nothing more than the accumulation of mutated cells. We have these kinds of cells in our system since the day we are born and are simply the leftovers of cell repair. When cells get old or damaged they are replaced by new and healthy cells. If your energy level is normal, which means your immune system works perfectly, it will eliminate these damaged cells and free radicals. We don't have to think about it and don't even need to do anything about it; it's just the normal way of life to replace old or damaged body cells with new ones.

In fact, every six weeks we have a brand new liver. That means if your liver is damaged today it does not need to be that way in six weeks. The entire body is replaced by cell renewal every seven years. The only cells that do not renew themselves are nerve cells, such as the brain cells. That isn't bad though because we know today that other brain parts can take over the work of damaged parts of the brain after a stroke, for example.

I'm telling you this because *The Only Answer to Cancer* is a book of hope, and I want you to understand that there is always hope, no matter how bad your health situation is right now.

If your energy level and therefore your immune level are high and normal, you don't have to worry about cell renewal or body repair or self-healing. If your energy level is low, I want you to know that there are many ways to strengthen it and gain back your health.

Case Study of Healing with IBMS™
Healing Cancer of the Liver

I have witnessed many incredible, miraculous and spontaneous recoveries with cancer patients. Judy, who had liver cancer, was one of my most impressive patients. She was in her early forties and was referred by a physician from Göttingen, Germany, who gave her a maximum of two months to live. Judy was in the final stages of liver cancer. She attended other people's seminars, and experimented with various esoteric healing methods. Nothing seemed to improve her health, and Judy desperately wanted to recover.

I noticed immediately that Judy had no short term goals, nor a future perspective. She lived with her elderly, sick mother, who was waiting for her approaching death. Judy felt lonely and empty inside. After our first discussion, I encouraged Judy to attend a six-hour intensive course at our IBMS™ training center in Steinberg, Germany.

At the center, Judy developed a future perspective based upon her personality and interests. This gave her hope and confidence. Judy was encouraged to imagine herself interacting with sympathetic and compassionate people, even with a potential partner. Until now, Judy had never thought like that before. Within a short time, Judy changed drastically. Life became exciting for Judy, as she uncovered lots of new possibilities and opportunities for growth. She moved out of her mother's apartment, took up hobbies and developed new interests, including music dancing lessons. Shortly thereafter, Judy started dating and met a wonderful man to share her life with. Judy's healing was incredibly fast and spontaneous. Her physician examined her twelve days after the IBMS™ training, and documented that Judy's cancer had already receded. After three and a half months, the doctor made the diagnosis that Judy was completely cured. Today, Judy looks radiant and energetic. Her liver cancer never resurfaced.

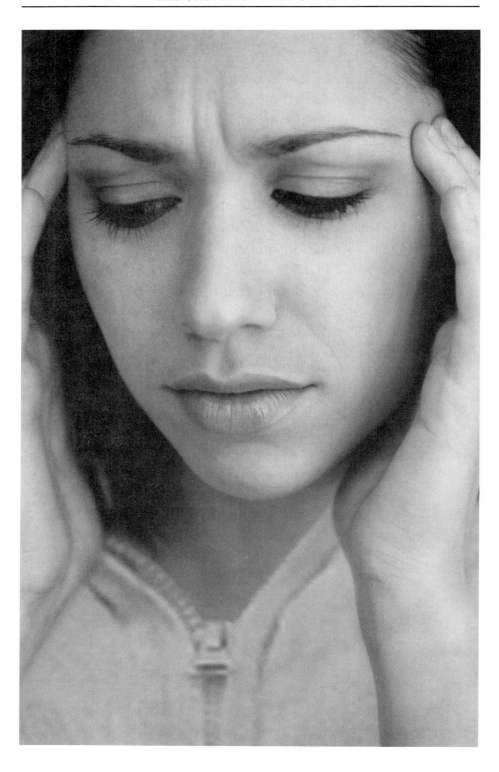

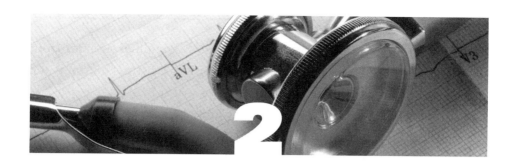

THE MAIN CAUSES
OF CANCER

The first cause of cancer is a lack of energy that debilitates the body's immune function, preventing it from doing its usual job. Once you're at this low energy level, it allows the damaged and dead cells to stay in the body and accumulate. They then start to replace new cells with their own damaged form and that accumulation becomes tumors which is called cancer. There are some tumors or cysts that grow and some do not. The dangerous ones are of course the growing ones, especially if they start to spread into the body and invade the surrounding body tissue.

These cancer cells need an acidic environment that lacks oxygen. Nobel Prize winners Otto Warburg and Max Planck received their Nobel prizes for proving that cancer cannot exist or grow in an oxygen rich and slightly alkaline (pH 7.36) environment. So was that not already the cure for cancer in 1936 when these facts were known and scientifically proven?

So, what causes an acidic body? Or, what puts it in a state of acidosis and a lack of oxygen? The answer is, first and foremost, *stress*! Nothing can make the body acidic faster than stress. Stress shuts down the metabolism so you can't get proper nutrition. Many illnesses stem from nutritional deficiencies which are actually caused by stress—even if the person has the best diet and nutrition in the world.

Stress truly does affect our health and well-being. Studies have shown that 86% of all illnesses are caused by stress, while a Stanford University study concluded that 95% of all illnesses are stress related! Even if we use the modest 86% figure, this means that only 14% of all illnesses are caused by other factors not related to stress.

The second cause of cancer is the accumulation of toxins in our system which mostly comes from our diet in one form or another. Fluoride and chlorine in our drinking water or toothpaste (just two teaspoons of fluoride toothpaste can kill you!), preservatives and taste enhancers, MSG, Aspartame (every artificial sweetener!), heavy metals and all of the countless toxins in vaccines and medications, prescriptions and over the counter drugs.

Other factors are malnutrition and microwaved foods, and the worst of all is milk! (See www.NotMilk.com) I would never drink milk since it will harm you in one way or another, plus the medications and anti-biotics and chemicals in milk can kill you if the milk doesn't do it. Did you know that milk is responsible for osteoporosis and most allergies, and also acne in teenagers?

If you've been diagnosed with cancer it's imperative to start on an organic, raw food diet. In fact, everyone should only eat organic foods. You also need to do a whole body cleanse twice a year to avoid the massive damage your body has to endure due to the accumulation of toxins. Twice a year I do the 21 day Be Pure full body and colon cleanse from www.MyBePure.com and the metal cleanse from www.HelpingAmericaNow.com. I take Quint-Essence and vitamins D and E, along with Flora-Zymes from www.AwesomeSupplements.com every day of my life, but, more on these later.

The third cause of acidosis and toxemia is a lack of hydration. Most people need at least a gallon of water a day with half a teaspoon of sea salt in it. Don't use table salt since it often has sand and/or glass in it which cuts your arteries and causes the accumulation of cholesterol to stop the internal bleeding. That's how you get high blood pressure! Use only sea salt or Stardust from www.GreatWholeFood.com.

For the best liquid nutrition and for those of you who do not want to swallow capsules go to www.trinisol.com

The fourth cause of cell damage is EMC (electromagnetic chaos) or EMF (electromagnetic frequencies). These are the damaging frequencies that come from cell phones, computers, microwaves, etc. We'll come back to this later, but if you want to know how to protect yourself best from these dangerous frequency waves go to: InstinctBasedMedicine@gmail.com or go to www.ewater.com

I've mentioned all of this so that you understand that a lack of energy, lack of oxygen in your body, and acidosis are caused by mostly controllable factors.

That means, if cancer can only live in an acidic and oxygen-lacking body, the cure or the way to the normal state of health is to change the factors that lead to acidosis, toxemia and lack of oxygen. Once you do this, your body goes back to its normal state of health!

Your Cancer Makes Them Rich

Now that you know how simple it can be to reverse the accumulation of mutated cells and get the body back to health, the next question is: Why isn't the medical profession using these scientific facts and simple truths to cure me of cancer?

As usual, the answer is always the same: Money! Money and power are the only true motivations of the pharmaceutical and medical industry. John D. Rockefeller needed sales people for the chemicals he produced so he created his own army of salesmen which we today call medical doctors. He started all of this insanity by creating and supplying education for medical doctors and controlling every aspect of medicine.

Poisoning the patient with a mainstream killer drug called Ifosfamide costs far over 10,000 dollars for a five day course. Plus you have to figure in the doctors and hospital fees, and the other drugs prescribed. The business of cancer brings them big bucks!

The McGill cancer center in Canada concluded after a secret study that 58 out of 64 oncologists said that all chemotherapy programs were unacceptable for their family members or themselves. They admitted that the drugs are ineffective and have an unacceptable degree of toxicity.

This statement from oncologist James Holland says it all: "My definition of cancer quackery is the deliberate misapplication of a diagnostic or treatment procedure in a patient with cancer … The culprit who victimizes his fellow man suffering from cancer … all the while greedily enriching himself, is a quack, a criminal, a jackal among men who deserves the scorn and ostracism of society. Because human life is at stake, he must be controlled." Of course, Holland has a different treatment plan that he applies to his patients.

As you can see, the trillion-dollar cancer industry is not interested in cancer cures, especially those that are fast, easy and natural. (In other words, not patentable!) Their publicized goal today is it to turn cancer into a manageable disease. Meaning, they make money off of the suffering of cancer patients even longer.

Cancer patients today usually do not die of cancer anymore, they die of the effects of the medical treatment of chemotherapy, radiation—which everyone knows causes cancer because who would want to live next to a nuclear reactor?—or surgery, which usually spreads the cancer throughout the system like an explosion. After they've caused cancer either through biopsy or surgery they call it a "fast growing cancer."

To damage an already weakened body that is cancer ridden with all these medications and medical procedures is absurd and is more like massive slaughter than anything.

Just go into the cancer division of a hospital and watch how healthy and normal most cancer patients look when they first arrive and then see how they look after just two or three treatments of chemotherapy. They usually look 10 or 15 years older within a few weeks. In fact, they almost look mummified. I personally have not been able to recognize patients that I knew after they had surgery and three chemotherapy treatments. I just passed by their beds because they didn't even resemble the person I had seen some weeks before.

Why Are They So Afraid?

Why is the medical profession, pharmaceutical industry, the FDA and others so afraid of people like me?

Because this book is capable of breaking down the power and trillion-dollar income source of the pharmaceutical and medical industry. Massive amounts of personal attacks, defamation, and lies against me will follow the publication of this book. But don't let this lead you to doubt my facts, proven successes and scientific facts that I have published in this book and the CD series that will follow. Always check www.InstinctBasedMedicine.com for the newest information.

Remember that they are the ones that make their money on our suffering, pain and death. And they use personal defamation or other illegal means as their main tool to silence opposition or competition. They attacked Kevin Trudeau personally for some stupidities and legal wrong doings he committed as a kid and made up more lies than I have ever seen directed at one person. They want to minimize and destroy the massive success Kevin has had with his book *Natural Cures They Don't Want You To Know About*!

To my knowledge, Kevin has sold over 50 million of his books and has educated the public about corruption, schemes, and the dangers of chemicals in food and drugs like nobody else before. Because he was right they could not attack the published facts, but they tried to destroy, defame and neutralize the person. I guess the same will happen to me.

So be warned, judge my book on the facts not on the lies and accusations they will throw my way. Listen to Kevin Trudeau's radio show at www.ktradionetwork.com because that will bother the criminals most.

I've already faced my share of assault. I have been shot at, my car has been bombed and I have been threatened, blackmailed and bribed to stop my work and just go away. As you see, I have 11 bestselling books in Europe, have had over 35,000 patients, 2.2 million seminar attendees, co-authored a couple of successful books in English, and my first book in English, *Instinct Based Medicine: How to Survive Your Illness and Your Doctor*, sells extremely well. In spite of these facts, the media does not support this book although it is already my publisher's mega-bestseller.

So when the trouble starts remember the facts. Two independent studies have concluded that I do have the highest cancer cure rate in the world (92.3%). I also cured my own mother from liver cancer in the terminal state over 30 year ago. Look at the countless cured cancer patients worldwide and not at the accusations and lies they come up with. They are also very good in creating "facts."

This has been enough space and time wasted on these crooks, let's get you healthy and focus on the positive things instead of the negative.

Preventing Cancer or Any Other Disease is Simple

By following these basic good health practices you'll save yourself much pain, suffering and money:

* Do regular cleanses every year

* Have a diet that consists of 70% good, healthy, living food

* Drink a gallon of good water every day

* Add some necessary supplementation—nutrient levels are not in sufficient amounts in our food anymore

* Get enough sleep

* Have some kind of minor but regular exercise routine such as walking half an hour a day, or using a rebounder (mini trampoline) for seven minutes twice a day

* Get at least 15 minutes of sun on your skin daily without sunscreen—sun does not cause cancer, it cures it

* Have a healthy attitude toward life

* Respect the basic laws of God and Nature

* Nutrition, oxygen, water, movement, regeneration, sleep, stress reduction and prevention will go a long way in keeping you healthy. But in case something goes wrong, you start feeling sick, tired or

worn out, instantly go to fresh juicing and doing the right things 100% of the time until you feel good again

By following my recommendations for a healthy lifestyle you should find yourself enjoying peak health and energy. But, if you ever get really sick because you violated the laws of God or Nature you need to do whatever it takes to "rehealth" yourself as quickly as possible. Of course, I suggest you look into my suggestion for Rehealthing!™ Rehealthing means using the magic of your own God or Nature given healing powers.

Cancer Is a Life Lesson

To discover and understand the physical causes of cancer, you will first need to let go of the idea that cancer is a powerful disease that must be fought. You never fight a symptom; you heal the carrier of the symptoms. You get what you focus on. If you focus on the cancer then you get more cancer. If you focus on health, that is what you get.

Healing is accepting, allowing and supporting, not fighting or resisting. Spontaneous remissions occur when the body can use its maximum healing capacity because it is not preoccupied with a fight or flight response situation caused by stress.

There is something to be learned from every situation, including having cancer. A person's willingness to face, accept and learn from the issues that cancer brings up could be the most important experience in someone's life.

There is always an underlying root cause of every situation, even if it seems unrelated. You, as consciousness or soul or spirit, are the only controller of that energy and the information that runs your body. Your presence in the body and what you do, eat, drink, feel and think determine how well your genes are able to control and sustain your physical existence.

Cancer can be a provider of new life. Cancer only strikes when a part or parts of us are not alive anymore; physically, emotionally, and spiritually. It usually goes hand in hand with a conscious or subconscious command that the person does not want to live any longer in these specific circumstances. Cancer can be a wakeup call so that you can look at and resurrect these numbed, suppressed, or congested areas, whether they are physical or non-physical in nature.

Cancer Is Not a Disease

The majority of the medical and lay population holds the belief that the gradual *degradation* of normal cells into cancer cells is due to random mistakes that the body somehow makes, perhaps because of hereditary reasons, often called genetic predisposition. This theory defies all logic.

These kinds of cancer cells are created every day to make certain that the immune system remains stimulated enough to keep its defense and self-purification capabilities efficient and up-to-date, plus it's a natural part of the body's cleansing process.

The cancer is not a disease but an extended immune response to help clear up an existing condition of congestion that suffocates a group of cells. Why would the immune system try to hinder the body's efforts to prevent this congestion? Cancer cells are far too precious and too useful for the body to eliminate them. Cancer cells do not randomly spread throughout the body. They lodge themselves in places that are also congested, places that are oxygen-deprived.

For example, it is similar to the fact that maggots eat only the desired part of a wound. If placed on someone's open, infected wound they don't eat the healthy tissue. Because of this, they are sometimes medically used for wound cleansing purposes. Bacteria are only found in diseased parts of the body. If you don't have toxic and poisoned parts in your body then no bacteria can grow and multiply. This means, if you have any kind of infection you know you have rotting or toxic parts in your body.

The Different Stages of Cancer

1. Blockages

Cancer begins when there is congestion in an area. Like a river that stops flowing, the water gets stagnant and toxic very fast.

2. The restriction of oxygen flow, dehydration and lack of nutrition to the cells

A restriction of oxygen flow can be generated by thickened blood vessel walls which prevent the proper passage of oxygen, water, glucose and other vital nutrients from the blood to the cells. This could be due to the consumption of red meat, smoking and trans-fats. Cancer and heart disease generally share the same physical causes. Even if the physical part of any disease is a maximum of 14% and 86% is stress related, these are a very important 14%.

3. Slow or blocked lymphatic flow

The lymphatic system is basically the main part of your physical immune system. The degree of nourishment, health and efficiency of the cells depends on how swiftly and completely waste material is removed through the lymphatic system. We have four times more lymph liquid than blood. But, unlike blood that has the heart as a pump, the lymph liquid does not move on its own and can only be moved by deep stomach breathing or aerobic exercise.

In my experience the lymph system is consistently blocked in cancer patients. My patients in Europe always got full body lymph drainages twice a day. If you ever visit Europe and get a full body lymph drainage, it will boost your health and immune function. I believe it is not available in the US.

4. Regular and frequent problems with digestion

Very often, before a person experiences chronic lymphatic congestion, they usually have long-term difficulties with digesting food. Improperly digested foods become a breeding ground for toxic compounds that can affect cellular behavior. Poisons like fluoride, chlorine, artificial sweeteners, vaccinations, other drugs and toxins are often the main cause of lymphatic blockage. But keep in mind that nothing can restrict or block body functions like stress.

5. **Liver function and bile duct flow restriction**

Gallstones are not only found in the gallbladder, but also in the bile ducts of the liver. Cancer patients and those suffering from arthritis, heart disease, liver disease, and other chronic illnesses, appear to have the most stones in their liver. Gallstones in the liver are the main obstacle to achieving and maintaining good health, youthfulness, and vitality. They are one of the major reasons people become ill and have difficulty recuperating from illnesses, including cancer. The main cause for gallbladder stones is stress.

Common Physical Causes of Cancer Cell Growth

- Unnatural foods and beverages, red meat and fried foods, preservatives, MSG, etc.

- Microwaved foods

- Cell phone and wireless devices, laptops and radiation.

- An increase in inflammation from gum disease can spread throughout the body, and there is a suspected connection between gum disease and cancer

- Sunglasses and sunscreens. These cause cancer because they don't allow the body to get enough ultraviolet light, which is one of the most powerful natural medicines in the world. Sunlight is proven to be a beneficial treatment of almost every type of illness and cancer. It can even eliminate skin cancer. It provides vitamin D and raises serotonin levels in the brain. Depressed people receive instant benefits from the sun.

- Toxic cosmetics and environmental poisons

- The most powerful direct and indirect causes of cancer are pharmaceutical drugs, cancer diagnostics and treatments such as mammograms, radiation, chemotherapy and surgery.

The Root Cause of Cancer: Emotions

The true root cause of cancer is a life of emotional negativity. Things like a lack of love or self-love, low self-esteem and a sense of worthlessness, living in constant doubts, worries, fears and living in compromises against yourself.

If you're in a relationship that you can't stand being in any longer or have a job that's killing you in every sense of the word, then *that* is what causes your cancer. Cancer can only exist in an environment lacking in energy. This must be an ongoing (chronic) form of lack of energy to be able to cause cancer. However, major emotional shocks can also be the trigger for cancer cells to develop.

Whatever happens in our emotional existence happens in our physical body. Cancer can come from just one trapped and isolated emotion, a feeling of having no choice, helplessness and hopelessness. Mind and body are connected, and any repressed feelings such as wanting and deserving love, acceptance, harmony, success, peace, stability, freedom, and a simple sense of joy in life are translated into appropriate biochemical responses in the body.

Whatever emotions or past traumas you keep to yourself out of fear of being criticized or laughed at actually turn into poisons in the body. But, the main problem is denial. What I mean by this is that subconsciously you know that something is really wrong and needs to change but you take no action to correct it. You continually make excuses or ignore it. Of course, not letting go of past traumatic events is another major root cause of cancer. My solution, instead of 15 years of Psychotherapy, is to simply get over it and move on!

Rejection or the Sense of Failure Can Cause Cancer

All events in life that appear to be negative are actually unique opportunities to grow as a human being and move forward in life. Whenever we need to give ourselves more love, joy, timeout, self-acceptance and appreciation, but fail to fulfill these essential needs, someone or something in our life will push us in that direction.

The human body is like the battery in your cell phone, no matter how good it is, it needs to be recharged regularly. The main problem is that people very often do not take enough time to regenerate and they burn out very fast.

Remember, the only cause of illness is a lack of energy and missing elements of rest, fun, happiness and the positive experiences that make life worth living and worth fighting for.

Feeling rejected by or being disappointed and angry with another person shows a lack of taking responsibility for the negative things that happen to us. Blaming oneself or someone else for an unfortunate situation results in the feeling of being a victim and is likely to manifest itself as disease. Moreover, if we cannot understand the messages behind our illness, we may even have to face death to appreciate living.

Make sure to recognize that opportunity and power lies within you. You need to accept the fact that you have a direct influence on your life, health and circumstances. You have the power to determine your individual level of health, happiness and your life circumstances! If you use this knowledge and power, all of a sudden your life will change and you will finally be in control.

As you can see, cancer can actually be viewed as a wake-up call to finally change your destructive life situations that paralyze you. It helps to break down old, rigid patterns of guilt, hate, fear, anger, unresolved issues of the past and the shame that keeps you imprisoned and bound by a constant sense of poor self-worth, lack of self-love or low self-esteem.

Have you ever heard of a person having a sudden heart attack and changing his life dramatically afterward because he now sees the value of life? The same often happens to cancer patients.

A Different Approach to Cancer

The current medical approaches don't target the root cause of cancer, but target only the disease process of cancer. Chemotherapy, radiation, and surgery encourage a victim-like mentality in the patient and are unlikely to heal the true cause of the disease. Cures that are considered miraculous only occur when a person becomes free of the need for victim-hood and self-destruction.

Furthermore, we need to love every part of our body, and accept who and what we truly are. We need to accept our own personality traits and characteristics and stop hiding parts of our self if we want to live in health and peace. Cutting pieces of your body out through surgery or destroying them with poisonous drugs or deadly radiation adds even more violence to your body than it already has to deal with. I have seen many cancer patients that hated themselves and their own body, and after the medical treatment they received did not even want to live anymore with all the deformation, damage and trauma.

If your friend or loved one has been diagnosed with cancer, to help them get through the disease process, allow them to experience the pain, despair, confusion, loneliness, hopelessness, anger, fear, guilt, and shame that they have been suppressing. If the afflicted person knows that he or she can express all these feelings without having to hide them, cancer can become a very powerful means of self-healing.

Cancer just alerts us to the fact that we are out of balance, and to cure ourselves we don't need to fight the cancer, we just need to get back in balance with ourselves and we will finally be healthy without having to do anything else.

Unresolved conflicts, living a life of self-denial, self-hate or constant compromises against ourselves are the starting points of any illness, including cancer. Cancer basically is the physical information letting the person know that he or she does not want to live in these negative life situations any longer.

Cancer Often Means Not Loving Yourself

A great number of people with cancer have devoted their entire lives to helping and supporting others. But, if the motivation behind it is to get love in return, it is an indication of not loving yourself. By taking care of and helping others this locks up unresolved issues, fears, and feelings of unworthiness, allowing the person to focus on someone else rather than their internal issues.

The Immune System in Action

Cancer always manifests as the result of an already toxic and acidic state in the body. It is not the cause but the *symptom* of ill health. Despite huge efforts and expenditures by the medical establishment, mortality rates from cancer have not decreased in over fifty years. In fact, the opposite is true.

Tumor cells are cells that "panic" due to a lack of food, water, oxygen and space. Survival is their basic genetic instinct, just as it is ours. Everyone believes that cancer cells are responsible for the death of a person; the whole medical system is based on this idea. But how is it then that most cancers just disappear on their own?

Cancer cells actually help a highly congested body survive a little longer than it would without them. It is part of a cleansing and survival mechanism. These cells are doing a critical job in a body that's filled with toxic waste. The cells don't randomly become poisonous or malignant; they do it to avoid an immediate catastrophe in the body. If the body dies, it is not because of cancer, but because of the underlying reasons that led up to it.

Tumors act like sponges for the poisons that circulate and accumulate in the blood, lymph and tissue fluids. These poisons are the real cancer, and they continue circulating unless a tumor filters them out. By destroying the tumor, the real cancer keeps circulating until there is a recurrence. Cancer is in the person not in body parts. Cancer is a mental and emotional illness with physical symptoms and always combined with or totally caused by stress.

Poisons such as chemotherapy drugs and antibiotics make the causes of cancer spread and become more aggressive. The tumor is an outlet for poisons. That is the reason why surgery often leads to an explosion of cancer cells in the body and a very fast death because the surgery sets the toxins free that would have been still locked up within the tumor before the surgery.

The human body is perfect and always pushing us toward health and wellbeing. We have survived all of these generations without chemical drugs and surgery or radiation and most of all vaccinations, and we certainly don't need it now.

Please be aware of the fact that so-called modern medicine is not even 100 years old, yet how old is mankind? Nature does not make mistakes; we are built to survive and to repair and to regenerate and to rehealth by getting back in balance. We are pure energy and if our frequency is in balance with who we really are, we are healthy, happy and successful.

The Body's Desperate Attempt to Survive

Cells only go into a defensive mode and turn malignant if they need to ensure their own survival, at least for as long as they can. A spontaneous remission occurs when cells no longer need to defend themselves. Nobel Prize winners Otto Warburg and Max Plank have scientifically proven that cancer cannot grow in and alkaline oxygen rich body. I also want to remind you that the body has to be acidic on a pH scale under seven (seven is neutral, below is acidic) and stress is the main cause of illness and decay because it causes acidosis.

Most cancers occur after a number of repeated warnings which may include:

- Headaches that you continually stop with pain killers

- Nausea, dizziness and lack of motivation

- Tiredness that you keep suppressing with a cup of coffee, tea, soda or energy drinks

- Nervousness you try to control through nicotine or sugar

- Medicines you take to ward off unwanted symptoms, such as from a cold or the flu

- Seasonal head colds or unidentified pains and symptoms

- Not giving yourself enough time to relax, laugh, and be quiet

- Conflicts you keep avoiding, living in denial or hating yourself or even life itself

- Pretending that you are always fine when you are not. Putting on a show is very energy draining

- Having a constant need to please others, while feeling unworthy and unloved by them

- Low self-confidence, low self-esteem or feelings of worthlessness that make you strive constantly to prove yourself to others

- Rewarding yourself with unhealthy comfort foods because you feel undeserving

- Numbing yourself with alcohol and drugs to avoid reality

Genetic mutation is the main physical cause of cancer; yet in truth it is only an effect of living in toxicity. Cancer is the final attempt of the body to live, and not, as most people assume, to die. Without gene mutation, those cells in the body that live in a toxic, anaerobic environment would simply suffocate and expire. In many cases cancer symptoms itself can be the cure.

Why Most Cancers Disappear Naturally
Scientific evidence suggests that most cancers disappear by themselves if left alone. Every toxicity crisis, from a complex cancer to a simple head cold, is actually a healing crisis that, when supported through cleansing, hydration and perfect nutrition can be healed.

Numerous researchers have reported over the years that various conditions such as typhoid fever, coma, menopause, pneumonia, chickenpox and even hemorrhage can spark a spontaneous remission of cancer. They remove large amounts of toxins and help the cells to "breathe" freely again. Even fever, sweat, loss of blood, mucus discharge, diarrhea, and vomiting can get rid of toxins as the immune system receives a much-needed boost.

This is why I developed a specific cleansing system for my patients that is fast, safe and effective. In my experience this system stops the cancer instantly in its tracks. But, because it has no apparent scientific basis, it isn't used for further cancer research. Cancer researchers will take no notice of natural cures; they are not trained or paid to do so because it doesn't bring in any money!

Illness is nothing more than the body's way of getting rid of trapped poisonous substances. Blocking the exit routes for these poisons, which happens when symptoms are treated, can suffocate the body and stop its vital functions. The body has an innate tendency and capacity to heal itself. True medical treatment should support the body without interfering with it.

You cannot get a full blown infection without having toxins and acid in your body first. The microbes need a toxic and acidic environment to multiply, but if your body has an alkaline pH level of 7.36, is detoxified and nutrient rich, no massive bacteria or virus infection is possible.

Other Causes of Cancer

The main outside cause of cancer is EMC (Electro Magnetic Chaos from cell phones, computers, etc.) and environmental poisons like fluoride or chlorine in drinking water, or food preservatives and artificial sweeteners such as aspartame.

Please see my website www.InstinctBasedMedicine.com to learn how to protect yourself from these dangers:

- The suppression of children's diseases through unnatural immunization programs can put the children at high risk for eventually developing cancer

- Wearing bras impair lymph drainage

- Early puberty and breast cancer link may be caused by rising childhood obesity rates, inactivity, and hormones in food

- Soy is a cancer- and disease-causing food

- French fries and other fried, baked or roasted carbohydrate-rich foods contain the chemical acryl amide

- Toxins contained in air pollution

- Microwave ovens. Overeating and excessive weight gain

- Watching television daily for several hours

- Not enough cholesterol (Again, you die of not enough cholesterol, not too much of it!)

- PVC shower-curtains, plastic water bottles and containers

- Artificial sweeteners such as Aspartame and Splenda

- Growth hormones in cow's milk

- Synthetic vitamins

- Grilling meat, poultry or fish

- High intake of fructose and sucrose

- Smoking cigarettes

- Sunscreens

- Night Shift Work

- Blood transfusions

- Chlorinated water

- Fluoride in municipal drinking water

- Wireless devices

- Pesticides and other chemical toxins

- Hair dye

- Arsenic, asbestos, and nickel

- Teflon

Dehydration Linked To Cancer

Cancer growth usually occurs in areas of severe dehydration. (Remember, the cause of all disease and illnesses is *stress*!) You need half a teaspoon of sea salt in a gallon of water each and every day to get and stay hydrated. Our cells can run dry for a number of reasons:

- Lack of water intake

- Consumption of beverages that have a diuretic effect like coffee, caffeinated tea, sodas, energy drinks, and alcohol

- Consumption of stimulating foods or substances such as meat, hot spices, sugar and tobacco

- Stress

- Most pharmacological drugs

- Excessive exercise

Routine Cancer Screening—Their Way to Recruit Patients

Cancer screenings are more sensitive than ever before, but since they don't have a cure, what in the world does early detection really do for you? Nothing!

Then we have breast self-examination. Women are urged to check themselves out once every month. Please, stop this self-diagnosis and of looking for cancerous lumps. The reason is because you will usually find what you are looking for! Besides, these harmless lumps or knots usually go away on their own if you give your body the chance.

It has been proven that all of the prostate cancer screenings in the past were harmful or at the very least worthless.

Mammograms have never been proven to prevent or cure cancer or to save or prolong the life of cancer patients. It's all a marketing scheme to make money on the diagnostics and to create customers. In my opinion, it has no realistic or scientifically proven value. My wife and mother would never be tricked into doing any of these murderous early detection frauds. I have more to say on this in the next section.

They try to make us believe that medicine is based on scientific facts, but if that were true, why would they have to change their opinions, conclusions and treatments every six months?

Mammograms Are Literally Squeezing The Life Out Of Women!

Professor Michael Baum of the University College Hospital in London states: "Thousands of women are being deceived by the national cancer program. They are led to believe that early detection of cancer will save their breasts. Half of the women with 'early' breast cancer are having mastectomies that might be later proven unnecessary. It is definitely a false promise that if due to some kind of screening the cancer is detected early and the woman's breast can be saved! "

The problem is that women with so called ductal carcinomas (small, localized, very confined lesions) usually require no treatment at all since they typically go away on their own. However, women are used to being misled and panicked into unnecessary mastectomies.

Mammograms may be able to activate an otherwise dormant and benign condition. I am sure mammograms *cause* cancer and I personally see no legitimate reason for them at all.

Instead, once a year do the IBMS™ cancer cleanse and you should be fine. In my experience, if patients have serious cancer tissue growths in their body they usually feel or know something is wrong. Even so, I believe there is still enough time to apply a natural cure! Don't be taken in by the medical profession because they have not found a reliable cure. They don't even know where cancer comes from. They only know how to diagnose cancerous tissues in the lab and how it usually behaves once they start to mess with it.

Every compression during a mammogram leads to microscopic ruptures of tissue, including the tumor tissue. This spreads the cancer and can lead to an early death. When the doctor manhandles a woman's breasts with hard pressure it can spread the cancer! The technician squeezes the woman's breast between the photographic plates with maximum compression that equals the weight of a 50 pound sandbag. Or, better said, they squeeze the life out of the women. If it hurts, it's wrong!

One animal study showed that manipulating a tumor increases the number of metastases by 80%, while a human study showed that women that had a mammogram have a 29% increased chance of dying of breast cancer than women who had never had one. My own grandmother had a cancerous tumor in her breast for 28 years. It did not grow or hurt in anyway and it did nothing until they did surgery on her and she started dying that very day.

Cancer is usually extremely slow growing and I have never seen an aggressive, vicious cancer occurring before they messed with it. It can take a cancerous tumor ten to twenty years to grow from the size of a pea to the size of a walnut. So what is the hurry or even the reason or benefit of fast surgery, chemo and radiation?

What's the benefit in giving up your quality of life? Plus, there are countless proven natural cancer cures available today. But, thanks to the FTC, FDA and ACS, many are not available in the USA.

Plus, the lymph system is the foundation of our physical immune system and the lymph nodes are the chemical neutralizers for the toxins in the body, how can it be helpful in any way to cut out these parts and impair the self-healing system even more?

If you regularly do breast self-examinations please know that if you feel a lump and it turns out to be malignant it isn't a death sentence and you don't have to lose your breast. Actress Christina Applegate opted for a double mastectomy because the medical community scared her. She believed that unless she had her breasts removed she would not have a very long life. In my opinion though, the more lymph nodes that are taken out, the shorter the lifespan. Of course, these are just my thoughts and I'm not a fortune teller. So far, my predictions have never been proven wrong.

Fast Facts about Mammograms:
• They have never been proven to prevent cancer or death

• Each x-ray you have done increases your risk of abnormal cell growth

• The National Cancer Institute (NCI) reports that among women under 35, mammograms could cause far more cases of breast cancer than it identifies

• A Canadian study found a 52 percent increase in breast cancer mortality in young women who had received annual mammograms

Prostate Cancer Screening—More Problems than It's Worth
Equal to the worthless mammogram line of attack against disease is the PSA screening (PSA Prostate Specific Antigen.) The PSA was supposed to determine if a patient has prostate cancer and how best to treat it. It is now proven that it does nothing except put money in the doctor's pocket. Even the JAMA essentially published:

A blood test to detect prostate cancer may lead to more problems than it is worth. The PSA test will lead many healthy men to undergo needless surgery for prostate cancer, damaging their quality of life while raising the country's medical bills.

Findings with the intervention in prostate cancer show that increased life expectancy after surgery was only 0.6 days for a 50-year-old man and 1.7 days for a man in his 70s. This is ridiculous! The patient experiences a tremendous loss of quality of life, incredible pain and suffering and impotence, just to gain 0.6 to 1.7 days? Do I really need to say more here to prove my point about the worthlessness of medical failures?

If you need more information though, how about this: There are at least 20% false positives with the test. Even Professor and MD Paul Frame of the Rochester School of Medicine and Dentistry said that clinical trials have not shown that the PSA test actually save lives.

So, let me ask again, what is the point?

Screening For Lung Cancer?

Dr. Stephen Swensen, chairman of the radiology department at the Mayo clinic, studied 1,520 smokers and former smokers. He found that 37 had cancer, but he also found that over 90% of them had unnatural cell growths. Also, over 2,800 had suspicious lung nodules and hard lumps ranging in size that was sometimes treated with surgery. It is speculated that most of the lumps or nodules would never have been found, nor would they have caused any kind of problem to the patients.

Our bodies are usually overloaded with some kind of junk anyway and if you don't do the recommended cleanses, such as the whole body cleanse I've been recommending from www.MyBePure.com once or twice a year, doctors will always find something to treat or cut out if they look for it. But, just because they do find something, it doesn't mean it will cause any harm or problems as long as they leave it alone. Most things will disappear on their own with regular cleanses, a healthy life-style and proper nutrition. If something looks suspicious to the oncologist, his eager surgical buddy will make some money! Swensen stated: *People who undergo spiral CT lung scans probably assume that this could save their lives but this is absolutely unproven.*

The medical mindset, the way I see it anyway, is this: *Everybody is sick; we just haven't found it yet!* I strongly believe that every medical intervention in regards to cancer enhances the odds of a medical disaster.

Pap Smears

Besides the crime of killing your daughters with Gardasil, the HPV vaccine, or at least making them sick and infertile, cervical cancer is actually nothing to fear. Fear the prevention and treatment, not the cancer!

Cervical cancer is relatively rare and there is no reason at all for any kind of pap smear! Plus poking around in a woman's body will cause infections and/or spread them. Besides, I fully believe that gynecology is a useless profession recently invented to make money on patients. How do you think women stayed alive and healthy 100 years ago before they invented the cash cow known as gynecology?

The doctor will not tell you that the millions of pap smears conducted did not lead to any kind of a reduced mortality from cervical cancer. So, besides unnecessary suffering and dying earlier, what is the purpose? What is even worse is that there is no proof that having a pap smear will decrease a woman's chances of dying from cervical cancer. The opposite is true. The follow-up procedure after an abnormal pap smear result is called a colposcopy. This can lead to infection, hemorrhage, cervical stenosis—a blockage of the passage from the uterus to the vagina—and an unnecessary hysterectomy. Of course, you have to make your own decisions about all of these procedures. After all, it's your body and you have to live with the consequences of your decisions and actions. I'm simply informing so that you can make logical choices.

Colonoscopy

This is yet another routine cancer screening that's dangerous to your health. Colonoscopies can lead to bleeding of the colon walls. The patient usually receives heavy drugs during the procedure which also has negative effects. Plus, the health value of colonoscopies is not scientifically proven. I see no use for it, nor do any of my colleagues. I would never do it and this procedure killed my father! A good colon cleanse after a full body cleanse twice a year should be enough protection.

So, that's my short opinion on this subject.

Case Study of Healing with IBMS™
Recovery from Breast Cancer

Tracy was an attractive, self-confident woman with an extremely stressful job. She had an abusive relationship with a man whom she dearly loved. Tracy could not bring herself to end the relationship, despite the fact that her dependency on this man was counterproductive and unhealthy emotionally.

When Tracy discovered a knot in her right breast, she visited a gynecologist who examined her with ultrasound. When the gynecologist wanted to X-ay Tracy, she went to another medical practitioner. He suspected that it was only a swollen lymph node, and gave her an injection. If the diagnosis was correct, the swelling would disappear.

When the knot remained, Tracy went to the hospital for an X-ray. The surgeon removed the knot as well as the surrounding tissue from the breast, and fifteen lymph nodes from her right armpit, two of which were malignant. She was told that an additional treatment with radiation and chemotherapy would prevent the cancer from spreading. When Tracy consulted her gynecologist, he recommended that she first take some time to recuperate from the stress of surgery. Intimidated and fearful, Tracy sought the advice of an alternative health practitioner, who suggested that her illness had a psychological cause. Finally, Tracy felt empowered to leave her abusive relationship with her boyfriend.

Tracy came to my center upon the referral of a friend who overcame breast cancer using my tools and techniques. Twice a week, Tracy strengthened her inner self by applying my IBMS™ technique. Additionally, Tracy received oxygen treatments and metabolism therapy with natural additives. Shortly thereafter, Tracy found a new boyfriend, as well as a less stressful job. After three months of therapy, Tracy completely recovered from breast cancer. She wrote me recently, resolving to never again compromise her values with an abusive relationship, which would induce stress and cause severe health problems.

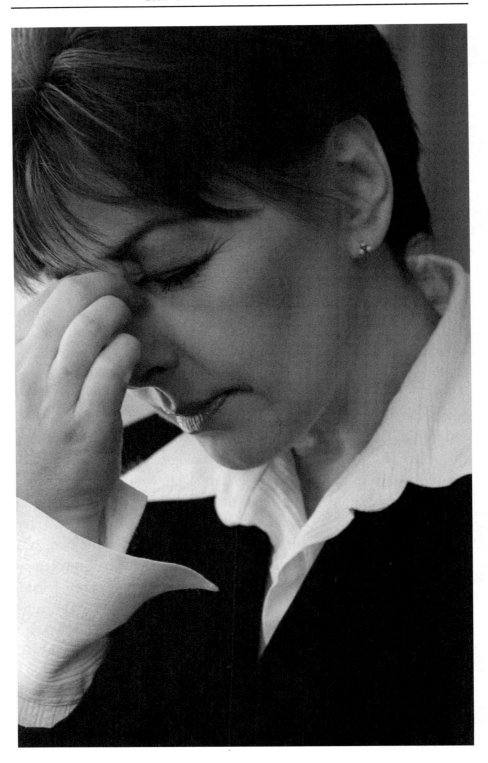

STRESS:
THE ROOT CAUSE OF
ALL DISEASES

The main tool I used in my clinics and healing centers in Europe was oxygen therapy. I found this to be the cheapest, fastest and safest way to produce health on all levels!

Oxygen is the most abundant element and the most crucial element in the human body and for life itself. For over 150 years oxygen therapy—or, in this case, Hydrogen Peroxide Therapy—has been used in Germany, Russia, Italy, Austria, and today in Mexico with huge success. It's now curing nearly every viral and microbial infection, even cancer, Multiple Sclerosis, Parkinson's and other deadly diseases.

The only reason why Americans have probably never heard of this fast and safe cure for cancer symptoms is the economic aspects. Basically, the power of the pharmaceutical industry because it costs about 2 cents a day to cure cancer with H2O2 (Hydrogen Peroxide). Compare that to the millions and millions of dollars they make through chemotherapy, radiation, and other drugs.

Of course there are the usual scare tactics from the pharmaceutical industry telling people Oxygen Therapy should not be used because of the dangers of oxidation. What many people do not know is that human cells are all surrounded by an enzyme coating which makes the cells resistant to oxidation. Viruses and bacteria and other disease-causing microorganisms do not have this enzyme coating and are therefore oxidized on contact with the application of hydrogen peroxide or ozone. If administered right it is in my experience that this is the safest and fastest way to cure cancer, AIDS, flu and all kinds of infections and diseases that are caused by infection.

Note: Please do not administer Hydrogen Peroxide before you have done your own research and have read the entire article and information on my website www.InstinctBasedMedicine.com. I believe, based on my use of oxygen therapy in different forms for over 15 years in my MTC® (Modern Therapy Centers™) that nothing is safer or more effective than bio-oxidative therapy if it is applied in the right form.

Prof. Dr. Manfred von Ardenne kept all the former Russian leaders alive and healthy for decades just with his Multi-Step Oxygen Therapy! After the fall of the Soviet Union when their leaders no longer had access to the Oxygen Therapy they literally died like flies in a very short amount of time.

In my MTC®s we used 35% food grade hydrogen peroxide diluted in 6 to 8 ounces of distilled water or aloe juice 3 times a day on an empty stomach—this is important or you may experience vomiting. We started with 3 drops 3 times a day (always diluted in 8 ounces of distilled water) and added one drop each day until we reached 25 drops 3 times per day for 35 days. We then started to cut down to 2 times a day and then once a day, while slowly getting down to 8 drops a day. As maintenance we used 8 drops of food grade 35% hydrogen peroxide in 8 ounces of distilled water three times day. It is highly toxic and can be even deadly if it is not diluted. It will even burn your skin. Never ever drink it undiluted!

In my centers we have seen massive cancer tumors shrinking within 14 days and that without any side effects. The success rate was nearly 100% and the hydrogen peroxide therapy gave hope to even terminal and late-stage cancer patients that were often just left to die by the medical profession.

As a reminder, oxygen or ozone therapy usually gets rid of all cancer symptoms quickly but it does not cure the cancer, it just eliminates the cancer symptoms, tumors and cancerous cells. Cancer is a systemic, mental and emotional disease and can only be cured if the root cause is eliminated. You have to find out what caused the mutation or tumor development and malignancy to spread in the first place.

Don't be fooled into believing if you find some elements or ways to manipulate your body—even with something like hydrogen peroxide—that you are cured because you are not! You have to uncover and eliminate the root cause of the cancer development or it will always come back, more vicious and stronger and faster than before. You cannot trick nature and pull yourself from the responsibility of eliminating the illness that you caused yourself in the first place.

Anyone who tells you that natural cures are dangerous or if they try to make them illegal or even access to them illegal should be jailed for life because he/she is a murderer in my opinion! Don't you think it should be a crime for the government or groups like the AMA, FTC, FDA, ACS, etc. to let you know that there are safe, effective and proven natural cures for cancer, AIDS, flu and more? And shouldn't they make them available to the general public? Instead, they do their best to keep the information and use of these natural cures out of our reach!

Doesn't this mean that they are indirectly responsible for the death of you or your loved one if cancer is the cause of that death and they know how it could have been cured easily and naturally?

If you don't fight with me, or at least support my fight for Patient Rights and Health Freedom as an Amendment to our Constitution and to stop the Banker owned Presidents and Government, you may not ever have the tools and elements available if you or your family members and friends may need them. Right now there are groups working to make the cures for cancer symptoms like Hydrogen Peroxide Treatments illegal and make the product inaccessible to us.

Stress is the Root Cause of All Diseases

Stress is the one major cause of acidosis. No matter what you eat or drink, if you have chronic stress then you have acidosis. In turn, this is the main, if not the only, physical cause of cancer, infection and illnesses of all kind.

In my opinion, mental and emotional stress is the root cause of all diseases, especially cancer! Stress can debilitate your immune system so profoundly that it no longer has the energy to sustain health. Every serious scientist and doctor recognizes the importance of stress in regards to health. The problem is that they have no idea what to do about it therefore they mention it and forget about it. Or, even worse, they prescribe drugs and numb the patient to a point where he is not able to fully function on a neurological level anymore. That does not help at all! That would be like having a splinter in your finger, but you don't look at or deal with the problem. Instead, you just push the splinter in deeper and take some pain and inflammation medication instead of pulling it out.

While oxygen is crucial for health and healing and prevention (which is why I invented the IBMS™ Session: Breathing Therapy) oxygen can only cure and support the body if the cells are able to receive the oxygen supplied by the blood. But, for the cells to be able to receive the oxygen they have to be open. If the cells are closed, such as from stress, they are unable to receive oxygen. This makes healing impossible and this is the main difference between the patients that get healed and the ones that did not.

As I just mentioned, the only cause for cells being unable to receive oxygen is stress. That is why stress, in my opinion, is the only cause for cancer—unless they radiate you to cancer and to eventual death!

Normally, all cells are under the control of the parasympathetic nervous system which controls the digestion of food, salivary gland secretion, blood flow to different parts of the body, and the absorption of nutrients. It is responsible for the proper function of the organs. While functioning under the parasympathetic nervous system, all cells are open, able to absorb oxygen and nutrients, get rid of waste products. They are healthy and dividing, multiplying, metabolizing and performing every task a cell needs to do to be a healthy normal cell.

When the cells are open they can absorb oxygen (you can usually feel it during my IBMS™ Breathing Session) and function properly. The body is easily able to heal itself. But, stress shuts down digestion and all other body functions.

The sympathetic nervous system gets activated by stress—either actual or perceived danger. The attack of a dangerous dog or an angry parent or spouse, are a few examples. Every negative emotion like fear, hatred, anxiety, worry or doubt can stimulate a stress response. Every negative memory or mental picture can cause stress.

Stress causes your autonomic nervous system to go into sympathetic mode and your blood flows away from your gastro-intestinal tract as well as from the skin. Your heart rate increases and your pupils dilate, the blood flows into the muscles and your body goes into high-alert mode. That is when the cells shut down! That is why chronic stress causes cancer—and nearly all other diseases.

If you live under chronic stress the body functions most of the time under the sympathetic instead of parasympathetic mode which causes, dehydration, nutritional deficiencies, lack of oxygen and acidosis—all of the physical causes of cancer and other diseases. That means the body functions primarily in the Fight or Flight mode and that causes many relationships to fail too.

Basically you can say that your state of mind is causing your stress and therefore your health or illness. It should no longer be a mystery as to why and how stress can kill! Stress is deadly, no matter what healing modality you choose. That is the true answer to the question why different people using the same treatment do not necessarily produce the same results.

What I see everywhere is that nearly every health author, every doctor or scientist, mentions the massive impact of stress in relation to health and illness. But instead of using the stress as a healing tool they just skip over offering a solution and instead recommend absurd, useless and often more damaging techniques like Mediation, Yoga, Hypnoses, NLP or other modalities. None of these will permanently reduce or eliminate the chronic stress in your life—I am absolutely sure about that! If you suppress stress it makes it even worse and living in denial can kill you. If stress is numbed by medication you will never be able to heal because you will not be able to address and eliminate the root cause of the life challenges that are causing your illness, unhappiness, lack of success, bad relationships and so on.

> Warning: Sometimes people eliminate the root cause of their stress and the second they feel better and are not afraid of dying anymore or the pain is gone, they go back to the stress caus-ing life situation and the cancer comes back faster, stronger and more aggressive than ever before. I have personally experienced that in most of these cases these patients died very fast after they got back into the cancer-causing life situation.

Remember that stress is not caused by external circumstances. Stress is caused by an individual interpretation of an internal image that causes the activation and takeover of the sympathetic nervous system and therefore the shutdown of the cells. That is what causes our cells to go into the Fight or Flight mode or, better said, into a state of self-protection. It is your individual response to an internal image (cellular memory) that determines your stress response.

My IBMS™ is created to help and teach you to deal with these stimuli in a healthy and positive way and to re-program your stimuli responses and to eliminate or recondition your internal interpretations and reactions. If you work with the IBMS Life Therapy™ (IBMS™ Healing Life Kit™) you will see and feel very fast everything I've been talking about! It is all about creating neurological pathways that you want and not just live with the ones that were created by life or coinci-dence and circumstance.

That is why a true stress reduction and prevention program has to include every form of personal development such as: goal setting, mo-tivation, health education, relationship, success, happiness education, training, and coaching. I am able to make all of this available and work-able to you with my Instinct Based Medicine® System™ (IBMS™). With my program you will experience positive results again and again!

You have to learn not to react to external circumstances; you have to be in control of your actions. However, you cannot be healthy if you don't feel successful in every part of life. That is why you should read my books: "You are born to win" or "The Success Guarantee" and use my IBMS™ audio system: Curing Life™. When you do, you'll get the essence of everything I have learned and taught in over three decades of research, therapy, training and coaching, in one simple to understand and easy to use system.

Stress reduction has to be so holistic that it includes every part of life

That is why I wrote so many bestselling books on different life issues. I wrote the most successful parenting book of all time in Europe, the most sought after book for sales people, books on relationships and every other part of life because all of this has to be included into one single system (IBMS™).

Yes, some people copy from other writers and practitioners and put all of these together and think it should work, but it doesn't. I truly believe that I have created a perfect system and I have many leading authorities backing me up on this. The reason is because I found the cure for cancer as a teenager and my results—not hypothetical statements—prove it. I developed the most successful motivational seminars and most sold book—*You Are Born To Win*—in Europe.

I also wrote the extremely successful book *The Sales Champion* and gave the most successful sales, management and personal development seminars in Europe. I trained and consulted for nearly all of the largest companies in Europe with unmatched success. I have over 2.2 million seminar attendees and over 35,000 patients that I got direct feedback from. I have over 7 million readers and millions of listeners to my program and radio shows and have gotten feedback from so many of them.

I have overcome countless diseases myself. I cured my mother and countless other people from cancer and can repeat this result any time! I had my own office at the age of 14 and was paying taxes. That is why

I am the best one to develop the only holistic system that really works to "Cure Life"™. My Instinct Based Medicine® system is and will be unmatched in success and results because life prepared me for this task for over 40 years!

I was the very first one who created the statement: "You have to eliminate the root cause of the disease or condition and then the illness and symptoms will disappear on their own." What bothers me most is the countless books and so-called experts saying that a single supplement, diet or subliminal audio program can get rid of the root cause of your disease. It can't! Disease is in your body, mind and spirit. It's in your mental and emotional world because we are simply all beings of energy living with the illusion of a physical body.

The only thing that can make us sick is if we violate God's or Nature's laws, and get out of balance, which then leads to an unhealthy energetic frequency. The absolute only way to "get rid of the root cause" is to cure life itself!

So, if you read anywhere that someone promises that you can get rid of the root cause of your individual health challenge by using supplements, herbs or any isolated technique, you can be sure that the person is not well-educated on the true cause of illnesses.

There is no magic bullet. There is no short cut. You made yourself sick over a long period of time and you are the only one that can fix the problem. And the problem is your entire life, not just one part of it. Except for accidents, all illnesses never come from one single source.

I hope that I can make you understand why I am so excited about this issue because it may harm you further or even kill you if you believe that there is only one single cause and one single solution for your heath challenges. You've been wasting valuable time and money, and hope and effort, all over a lie.

It's like chiropractics, which I believe in and love, but it does not get rid of the root cause of your back pain! You need to get rid of the stress that tenses up your muscles and pulls your vertebrae out of line so that you can heal. It gives you nothing but a short period of less pain but not a final solution. Many chiropractors now use my CD system in their offices to handle this problem for their patients.

I strongly believe that everybody can be cured from anything and that the only way to lifelong health is to create happiness and success, to live as your true self and your true personality, to develop and grow as a human being on a consistent basis, and to take charge and responsibility of your own life, your health and your future.

This is what I give you with my Instinct Based Medicine® System. I'm providing you with the education and the tools, the training and coaching to Cure Life™! This is the only answer to cancer, the absolute answer to any disease or condition. You have to use all the success producing elements that are available to you, learn all you can, follow various techniques or whatever you choose and use it.

That is how the medical profession misleads and tricks the public, they talk about hypothetical results based on statistics that are fraudulent to begin with and make up what they believe the results could or should be. And they are always wrong! Just look at the results that they are producing. They are losing the battle with every illness, most of all with cancer. Even with all the billions thrown into their research that has made them rich, they have done nothing to find the cure for cancer! With all that money, why are they still using primitive "cures" like radiation and chemotherapy?

That is why I beg you, if you have any doubts or when they start attacking me personally and try to discredit me with lies and defamation campaigns, look at my results: I cured my own mother from liver cancer and have, as concluded in two independent studies, the highest cancer cure rate in the world. And I can prove again and again that every cancer can be cured within 2 to 16 weeks.

So why does the government not give me the legal authority to personally practice my IBMS™ in the US and let me show them that I can help nearly everybody, as long as they have not had "traditional" cancer treatments yet?

Help and support me actively in my fight for a Constitutional amendment to Health Freedom and Patient Rights and all of us will be safer, healthier, happier and have a longer, more fulfilled life.

The Consequences of Stress

Stress leads to:

- Drug and alcohol abuse

- Self destructive behavior

- Toxemia—and diseases and pain

- Constricts muscles

- Is the leading cause for Acidosis—the foundation of poor health and all degenerative diseases

- Bad Relationships

- Physical malfunctions

- Sexual problems

- Lack of oxygen and dehydration

- Shuts down the metabolism and all body and neurological functions in part or as a whole

- Stress is the basis of every disease or disorder. In fact, in physics stress literally means: Pressure from the inside out

- Produces potentially harmful hormones such as cortisol and adrenalin which leads to an often unhealthy reaction to the fight or flight response

- Leads to nutritional deficiencies and obesity. It shuts down the metabolism and digestive system, and is the basis for all degenerative conditions, pain and pre-aging

- It depletes vitamins and hormones in the body

- Harms serotonin and melatonin production and

- Destroys vitamin B6 and zinc—needed for serotonin production

Stress Leads to Mental and Emotional Disorders Like:

- Depression

- Anxiety

- Frustration

- Hopelessness

- Lack of self-confidence, low self-esteem and lack of willpower

For licensed IBMS™ professionals, workshops and seminars or for education as an IBMS™ Practitioner, Therapist or Coach please go to: www.InstinctBasedMedicine.com

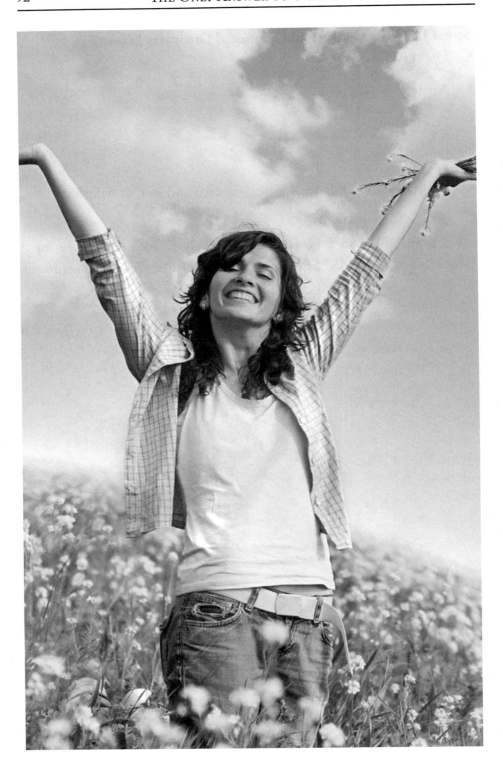

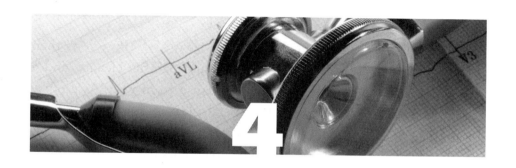

HOW TO PROTECT YOURSELF FROM CANCER

I know you're eager to find out how you can avoid getting cancer and many other diseases. You want to live a long, healthy, happy and successful life. Well, the good news is, you can! Of course, you've got to make some changes in your life. There's no way you can keep doing the harmful things to your mind, body, and emotions that you have been and expect to live in peak health.

This is what I've used over the years. It's a brief preview of the protocol I would recommend to anyone I know and care about. Later in the book I'll go more into detail. For now, I want you to get an idea of just how truly easy it can be to not only avoid getting cancer, but feeling better than you ever have.

1. First, get my IBMS™ stress reduction and self-help CDs. For more information go to my website: www.InstinctBasedMedicine.com. Without effective stress reduction, trauma relief and enhanced energy, the body cannot heal.

2. Diet and Herbs: I believe that if you eat only foods from www.GreatWholeFood.com and drink only filtered water and organic fresh juices you will become healthy no matter what your current physical health symptoms and challenges are.

3. Do a full body and colon cleanse from www.MyBePure.com, then a liver and gallbladder flush, Candida and parasite cleanse, and a kidney, lymphatic, lung and spleen cleanse from www.Awesome-Supplements.com. Also do the metal cleanse from www.HelpingAmericaNow.com. From www.UniversalFormulas.com get their life enhancing and life sustaining supplements like Quint-Essence, vitamin E, D and Flora-Zymes.

4. Eat plenty of fruits and vegetables that have cancer-curing and cancer-preventive properties such as Brussels sprouts, kale and cabbage. Most important is fresh juicing.

5. Take anti-cancer herbs including aloe vera, cat's claw, black cohosh, schizandra, and astragalus.

Try some of these helpful activities:

- Massage
- Art therapy
- Music therapy
- Dance therapy
- Physical exercise, ideally in natural light
- Breathing Therapy
- Biofeedback
- Other anti-cancer practices:
- Get plenty of sunlight (Sun cures cancer, it does not cause it.)
- Get plenty of sleep
- Eat regular meals
- Eat a vegan or vegetarian diet
- Get regular exercise
- Anti-cancer products that may be more effective than chemo
- Graviola
- Miracle Mineral Supplement

- Ojibwa Herb Tea-8-Herb Essiac
- A bicarbonate and maple syrup cleanse
- Marine phytoplankton

We will come to the true cures and healing later in this book, I just wanted you to get more familiar with this concept before we go into the details of the true and only cure for a person's individual cancer. I will explain cancer and cancer cures from different points of view and in different steps so that you get a holistic understanding for cancer and its cure.

Simple Ways to Reduce Your Cancer Risk

- Eat a variety of foods. Many foods contain protective substances-some that researchers are still discovering. And, getting nutrients from a varied, balanced diet will prevent you from getting too much of a potentially harmful substance.

- Eat more fruits and vegetables at least three servings of vegetables and two servings of fruits daily. Think color; deep green and yellow orange.

- Choose high-fiber foods. Besides fresh fruits and vegetables, add more whole grain breads and cereals and legumes (dried peas and beans) to your diet.

- Control your weight-avoid obesity. Keep an acceptable weight by eating moderately, limiting fats and sugars, and exercising regularly. Avoid diet and exercise extremes. Have a checkup before beginning a strenuous exercise program.

- If you drink alcohol, cut back. More than two alcoholic drinks per day puts you at risk for developing certain types of cancer, especially if you drink and smoke.

- Stop smoking, if you smoke, or don't start. Smoking is clearly linked to lung cancer. Chewing tobacco, snuff and pipes also cause cancer.

- Eat less fat. "Lean" toward low-fat meat, poultry and dairy foods, watch the high-fat snacks and desserts, salad dressings, etc., and bake, broil, stir-fry or steam-don't fry foods or add fatty extras.

• Limit highly salted, pickled and smoked foods, including charcoaled, grilled or broiled meats, fish and poultry.

Facts About Cancer and its Treatment

1. Every person has cancer cells in the body. These cancer cells do not show up in the standard tests until they have multiplied to a few billion. When doctors tell cancer patients that there are no more cancer cells in their bodies after treatment, it just means the tests are unable to detect the cancer cells because they have not reached the detectable size.

2. Cancer cells occur between 6 to more than 10 times in a person's lifetime.

3. When the person's immune system is strong the cancer cells will be destroyed and prevented from multiplying and forming tumors.

4. When a person has cancer it indicates the person has multiple nutritional deficiencies. These could be due to genetic, environmental, food and lifestyle factors.

5. To overcome the multiple nutritional deficiencies, changing diet and including supplements will strengthen the immune system.

6. Chemotherapy involves poisoning the rapidly-growing cancer cells and also destroys rapidly-growing healthy cells in the bone marrow, gastrointestinal tract etc, and can cause organ damage, like liver, kidneys, heart, lungs etc.

7. Radiation, while destroying cancer cells also burns, scars and damages healthy cells, tissues and organs.

8. Initial treatment with chemotherapy and radiation will often reduce tumor size. However prolonged use of chemotherapy and radiation do not result in more tumor destruction.

9. When the body has too much toxic burden from chemotherapy and radiation the immune system is either compromised or destroyed, hence the person can succumb to various kinds of infections and complications.

10. Chemotherapy and radiation can cause cancer cells to mutate and become resistant and difficult to destroy. Surgery can also cause cancer cells to spread to other sites.

11. An effective way to battle cancer is to starve the cancer cells by not feeding it with the foods it needs to multiply.
   Cancer Cells feed on:

   a. Sugar is a cancer-feeder. By cutting off sugar it cuts off one important food supply to the cancer cells.. Sugar substitutes like NutraSweet, Equal, Spoonful, etc are made with Aspartame and it is harmful. A better natural substitute would be Manuka honey or molasses but only in very small amounts. Table salt has a chemical added to make it white in color. Better alternative is Bragg's aminos or sea salt. The best of the best are the products from www.justlikesugarinc.com nothing is better and healthier as sweetener.

   b. Milk causes the body to produce mucus, especially in the gastrointestinal tract. Cancer feeds on mucus. By cutting off milk and substituting with unsweetened soy milk cancer cells are being starved.

   c. Cancer cells thrive in an acid environment. A meat-based diet is acidic and it is best to eat fish, and a little chicken rather than beef or pork. Meat also contains livestock antibiotics, growth hormones and parasites, which are all harmful, especially to people with cancer.

d. A diet made of 80% fresh vegetables and juice, whole grains, seeds, nuts and a little fruits help put the body into an alkaline environment. About 20% can be from cooked food including beans. Fresh vegetable juices provide live enzymes that are easily absorbed and reach down to cellular levels within 15 minutes to nourish and enhance growth of healthy cells. To obtain live enzymes for building healthy cells try and drink fresh vegetable juice (most vegetables including bean sprouts) and eat some raw vegetables 2 or 3 times a day. Enzymes are destroyed at temperatures of 104 degrees F (40 degrees C).

e. Avoid coffee, tea, and chocolate, which have high caffeine. Green tea is a better alternative and has cancer fighting properties. Water-best to drink purified water, or filtered, to avoid known toxins and heavy metals in tap water. Distilled water is acidic, avoid it. But 3 cups of coffee are okay in my opinion

12. Meat protein is difficult to digest and requires a lot of digestive enzymes. Undigested meat remaining in the intestines becomes putrefied and leads to more toxic buildup.

13. Cancer cell walls have a tough protein covering. By refraining from or eating less meat it frees more enzymes to attack the protein walls of cancer cells and allows the body's killer cells to destroy the cancer cells.

14. Some supplements build up the immune system (IP6, Flor-essence, Essiac, anti-oxidants, vitamins, minerals, EFAs etc.) to enable the body's own killer cells to destroy cancer cells. Other supplements like vitamin E are known to cause apoptosis, or programmed cell

death, the body's normal method of disposing of damaged, unwanted, or unneeded cells.

15. Cancer is a disease of the mind, body, and spirit. A proactive and positive spirit will help the cancer warrior be a survivor. Anger, unforgiveness and bitterness put the body into a stressful and acidic environment. Learn to have a loving and forgiving spirit. Learn to relax and enjoy life. In the opinion of over 2.2 million customers worldwide: " Nothing is more effective and helpful in this arena then Dr. Coldwell's Audio CD system.
See info at www.instinctbasedmedicine.com

16. Cancer cells cannot thrive in an oxygenated environment. Exercising daily, and deep breathing help to get more oxygen down to the cellular level. Oxygen therapy is another means employed to destroy cancer cells.

17. (My point) I suggest: 10 000 IU of Vitamin D 3 a day, vitamin C and E as well as quint essence and flora zymes from www.awesome-supplements.com to all my loved ones for cancer prevention and once a year the Cleansing system from www.mybepure.com and the metal cleanse and silver from www.healpingamericanow.com. Use only shampoo and soap and salt from www.greatwholefood.com and the only sweetener you should use is from www.justlike-sugarinc.com. Get as much sun as you can without sun screen and without getting burned of course. Plus, to avoid any further toxification from cancer causing fluoride and chlorine in your tap water, use the filters from www.ewater.com and to protect yourself from electromagnetic chaos get the EP 2 Pendant and cell phone booster, also from www.ewater.com

18. Instead of sugar or artificial sweetener get: Just Like Sugar from www.justlikesugarinc.com

19. No plastic containers in micro.

20. No water bottles in freezer.

21. No plastic wrap in microwave.

What You Focus On Expands

He who finds purpose and meaning in the occurrence of a cancer will also find the way to cure it. Tracing a cancer back to its origins is the key to true healing. Make sure you don't use cancer as a way to attract attention, to get pity, or (false) love.

Tumors of any kind are direct manifestations of negative emotions such as fear. Fear is synonymous with separation and defensiveness, constantly triggering the fight or flight response and draining energy. Resistance to cancer cells keeps a person in that state.

Whatever you focus on expands. It does not matter if you focus on fighting cancer or health; you get what you think about most of the time. Cancer cells heal spontaneously when your resistance disappears and you are able to replace this attitude with one of acceptance and love. When you consciously accept and embrace your resistances, you will not only lose the fear, but the body's cells can return to their natural balance and health.

Cleansing, pampering and nourishing the body are acts of accepting responsibility for what is happening to you and help you to become in control of your body and life. Show yourself how important you and your body are by treating it like the most valuable treasure in the world, because that is what you are.

Taking your power back and letting go of external crutches like suppressive drugs, aggressive treatments, and surgery are essential for healing your body, mind, and emotions. It is your body, your life, your future, your health. Your life is the result of your decisions and actions—nothing else.

We Are Created By Our Thoughts!

We are all built from atoms. If you could look into an atom you would see it is empty. That means we are built out of nothing. Or, better said, we are *pure energy*. According to the laws of quantum physics, in any scientific experiment the observer (a researcher or even yourself) influences and alters the object of observation on a very fundamental level. This applies to the human body as well, as it is composed of energy and information. Although something may appear to be solid, it is only perception that makes it appear so. Everything at the core is just energy and therefore dependant on specific frequencies.

Your thoughts are energy which influences other forms of energy, including the cells of your body. That is why the following statement is true: If you believe you can do something (like heal from or die of cancer) or you believe you cannot do it, you are always right. Your thoughts create your realty. You are what you think or believe you are.

If you believe strongly enough that you have cancer or if you are afraid of it, you face a significant risk of manifesting it in your body. The reason is that you manifest what you think about most of the time no matter if you are afraid of it or would love it. *What you think about most of the time becomes your reality.*

Chemotherapy: The Systematic Toxification of Your Body

Chemotherapy is so poisonous that leaking a few drops of the drug onto your hand can severely burn it. Spilling any chemotherapeutic drug in the hospital is classified as a major biohazard that requires specialists with spacesuits to dispose of it. Just imagine the holes chemotherapy creates inside blood vessels, lymphatic ducts, and organ tissues when you undergo infusion after infusion!

If your spouse is on chemotherapy you are advised not to be in physical contact with him or her, and after just one session of chemotherapy you are no longer allowed to be an organ donor. Chemotherapy can make you sterile and may also cause impotence.

The methods of modern or, better yet, *archaic* medicine, don't fight diseases, they fight the body. Often, disease is the body's way of healing itself, and modern treatment is a sure way to impair or even destroy this ability. Cancer patients don't usually die from the cancer, but from the symptoms of the "standard, law enforced medical treatment."

Scientists and medical doctors like Dr. Hamer and his "New Germanian Medicine" believe that cancer is not a disease, but a survival mechanism of the body designed to remove toxins that are causing harm. If so, would it not make more sense to support the body in its natural drive to remove such obstructions rather than to suppress its effort with aggressive, destructive means? I believe that it is always absurd to attack a symptom by harming the body. That makes absolutely no sense to irritate the immune system even further if the body is already in major distress.

Taking Responsibility for Your Health

Most people in the Western world turn to a doctor for every little problem they have. No one seems to want to take responsibility for their own life and health anymore. The food and medical industries have been manipulated for profit, power and control. Today, the masses no longer think for themselves and have lost common sense when it comes to their instincts for natural healing ability. They turn to an industry that has no interest in keeping them healthy and can only benefit when as many people as possible get and stay sick.

Many natural cures for cancer symptoms exist, and several are able to eliminate tumors or reverse unnatural cell growth, but none of them are being researched, endorsed, or promoted by those who claim to be the health custodians of the nation. The American Cancer Society, the National Cancer Institute, the American Medical Association (AMA), the Food and Drug Administration (FDA), and the major oncology centers all feel threatened by the successes of alternative cancer therapies.

That is one of the main reasons why natural cancer cures are suppressed and the scientists and therapists that uncover and successfully practice natural treatments and cures for cancer are destroyed, jailed, somehow "commit suicide" or "die of a sudden heart attack" without having had any heart condition before.

Usually, the founders and users of safe and effective natural cancer cures were ridiculed or ignored. If that didn't work, they were sued criminally and/or civilly until they gave up, went away, were financially ruined, or illegally put into jail.

My legal department stated that: *Nearly all of these convictions are illegal and go in line with false arrest, kidnapping, illegal detention, etc.*

And, the opinion of my legal department is: *The constitution is the supreme law of the land and any law, regulation, code or restriction made that is not in line with the constitution of the United States of America, is illegal, not valid and should not be held up in court as law.*

A solution to cancer would mean the end of many parts of the pharmaceutical and medical industry that "treat" and "research" cancer because cancer creates money and power for so many. Therefore, the criminals in these fields believe: Natural therapies must be disbelieved, denied, discouraged and disallowed at all costs, and all practitioners who are using these safe and effective procedures need to be destroyed or eliminated in any possible way.

Since the pharmaceutical industry owns and controls the media it is so easy to destroy someone's reputation or life, and defame all natural treatments as worthless or dangerous. And, since they own many, if not all, of the law making politicians, it seems to be obvious why so many unnatural, health endangering, health destroying and health killing laws are created—to protect the pharmaceutical industry and to further their profits.

According to independent reports by the prestigious *New England Journal of Medicine,* a wing of the American Congress, and the World Health Organization (WHO), 85-90% of all medical procedures used by today's medical establishment are unproved and not backed up by scientific research. Today's so-called modern medicine is therefore a religion and not a science because it is based on belief and not on science.

The symptom-oriented approach to treating disease generates a tremendous number of potential symptomatic side effects that, in turn, require further treatment. Even while they unsuccessfully treat one condition, they have already created the next ones. That is really conducting perfect business! But do we want our health and life to be a part of someone else's business?

It is not in the best interest of the medical industry, including the pharmaceutical companies, to find a real cure for cancer or for any other chronic illnesses, because this would make the treatment of disease symptoms obsolete.

At least 900,000 people die each year in the United States alone because of side effects caused by these symptom-suppressing and symptom-alleviating approaches. Pleases read my book: *Instinct Based Medicine—How to Survive Your Illness and Your Doctor*, to see all of the relevant the facts and statistics.

This is not to say that this trend is entirely the fault of the medical system, because the major part of the fault lies within the pharmaceutical industry that created the MD as their salesperson. The medical doctor is indoctrinated from day one in the study of medicine and later every single day by the pharmaceutical reps. People need to wake up before these industries kill them, their children and loved ones. People must take responsibility for themselves and for their physical and emotional health or the ones that profit from their suffering will do it for them.

Medically Treating Cancer Instead of Treating the Patient

Many people don't actually experience any symptoms until they begin medical cancer treatment. They soon lose their hair, their skin turns gray, their voice goes hoarse and they feel ill and fatigued. Their fingernails rot away and so do their gums until they lose their teeth. Vomiting, major pain, dizziness and nausea are only the tip of the iceberg of the effects of the so-called medical treatments. So what do your instincts tell you about these effects of the treatment? And by the way, these are the symptoms of the treatment not the side-effects. That is what these poisons do!

In 1990, German epidemiologist Dr. Ulrich Abel from the Tumor Clinic of the University of Heidelberg comprehensively investigated every major clinical study on chemotherapy drugs from 350 medical centers. He also reviewed and analyzed thousands of scientific articles published in the most prestigious medical journals. Abel's data was published in *Biomedicine and Pharmacotherapy* in 1992 and concluded that there is no scientific evidence available in any existing study to show that chemotherapy can "extend in any appreciable way the lives of patients suffering from the most common organic cancers." I'd also like to add that there are no scientific facts and physical results that can prove that chemotherapy ever cured a patient or prevented the patient's death.

Many doctors go as far as prescribing chemotherapy drugs to patients for malignancies that are far too advanced for surgery, with the full knowledge that there are no benefits at all since it achieves a 50% or more reduction in tumor size for 28 days. Temporary tumor shrinkage through chemotherapy has never been shown to cure cancer or to extend life.

Again, Chemotherapy has never been shown to have curative effects for cancer.

By contrast, the body can heal itself. Cancer is seen by some experts as a healing response rather than a disease. The disease in the body is caused by an existing imbalance. This healing response may continue even if a person is subjected to chemotherapy (and/or radiation). Unfortunately, the chances for a real cure are greatly reduced when patients are treated with chemotherapy drugs.

The effects of the treatment can be horrendous and heartbreaking for both patients and their loved ones, far more than the side-effects of the cancer.

Before committing themselves to being poisoned, cancer patients need to question their doctors and ask them to produce the research or evidence that shrinking a tumor actually translates to any increase in survival. Most of all, I urge you to speak to cancer patients that have been cured and that are still alive a decade or more later. Ask for physical evidence and proof that this "treatment" can cure you and that it has cured countless other people before.

Please educate yourself and you will learn that every effective natural treatment for cancer symptoms is more effective than all other medical treatments put together. Natural treatments have true cures and healings to show, while the medical treatments have none.

In mid 2009 a judge ordered a young boy, Daniel Hauser, to have chemotherapy against his will and the will of his parents who were seeking natural treatments. If I had a young child and a judge tried to murder him or her by ordering chemotherapy or any other form of homicide, I would seek legal actions against the doctor. Believe me, if I or someone I love were to be assaulted with any form of deadly force, I would use my legal right of self-defense to the fullest—and I mean to the fullest extent!

Protect Yourself Naturally

I'm convinced that all of these diagnostics in regards of finding cancer or diagnosing cancer are absurd. You don't even need to know if you have cancer or not. If you are in doubt just do a natural cancer treatment (see further information in this book) that usually has no side effects at all but eliminates the cancer symptoms, the tumor or cell mutation, and growth of cancerous cells.

Even if you don't have cancer it does not harm you at all, and you'll have a healthier body afterwards. Everybody should do a once a year general "rehealthing" protocol as I describe later in the book. It slows down or even reverses the aging process and usually gets rid of every malfunction, toxemia and acidosis in the body. You'll feel better, look younger, feel stronger and healthier, and have more energy, vitality and quality of life.

Even if you did not have cancer in the first place, the main outcome is that you will feel better and healthier. But if you have cancer and get chemotherapy, surgery or radiation therapy, you are damaged for life!

Cancer is not a disease, it is the final and most desperate survival mechanism the body has. It only takes control of the body when all other measures of self-preservation have failed.

They Think They Can Cure Cancer

I am so tired of people announcing that they have invented a natural cure for cancer then use this information to publish a book. In truth, I already published this information when I was 17 years old in my books: *Finally Say Goodbye to Your Illness* and *Mother Please Don't Die*.

Of course, there are over 300 cures out there that eliminate tumors and other mutations, but that does not mean the cancer is cured at all. It always comes back because treating or eliminating the tumor or abnormal cell growth or any kind of mutation does not cure the cancer at all. Cancer is systemic and caused by mental and emotional stress and the lack of energy caused by these forms of stress.

As long as you don't define and eliminate the root cause of your individual cancer there is no cure! After you have identified the main cause of your personal cancer development—such as living in constant fear, worries, doubts, compromises against yourself, lack of hope or goals, low self-esteem or self-confidence, unhappiness, lack of success, poor quality of life, or pessimism about your future—you will never permanently eliminate your cancer.

The subconscious mind constantly gets the order: "This body and mind does not want to exist any longer under these circumstances and these conditions." It does what you indirectly order it to do. Your subconscious will do all it can to take you out of the life situation that you do not want to live in any longer.

Of course, we don't consciously think about this, but it's a mute order directed at the immune system and the life sustaining systems. Often a divorce, loss of a loved one through death, bankruptcy, or other traumatic events can trigger the self-destructive order to eliminate your body. In other words, it will do all it can to get it out of the unbearable life situation or circumstances that you experience as unbearable.

After you have defined what life circumstances lead to this unconscious suicide, you have to get rid of the root cause of your health breakdown. Only then will the symptoms, tumors, and mutated cells disappear on their own.

Please remember that only 14% of all illnesses are caused by poor nutrition, dehydration, and lack of exercise. The truth is that 86% of the illnesses we face daily are caused by stress. Though this is certainly a very important 14%, it does not really matter in the long run because that is not the root cause of your cancer, it is only the physical by product.

What I am saying is even if you use all the proven cancer cures but don't eliminate the mental and emotional stress that leads to the lack of energy that leads to the health breakdown (cancer in this case) then there is no way you can you achieve any long-term result.

The only cause of illness is an ongoing or massive lack of energy; usually caused by mental and emotional stress such as living in fear, doubt and worry, not achieving your true potential, being someone other than yourself, and leaving behind your desires or dreams. The only reason for living is for personal growth and development, and if we don't grow as a person we feel unsatisfied and unhappy. The main problem is if we don't grow consciously then life makes us grow whether we like it or not, and that usually happens though illness, dissatisfaction, unhappiness, and negative life developments. It's better to choose your own way of growing than to let life pick something that ultimately makes you change or take action.

The Only Way to Be Cured

There are no incurable diseases only incurable people. These are people who are not willing to take responsibility and take charge over their own lives. Many are not willing to accept that they have made themselves sick and therefore cannot understand that they are the only ones who can cure them. They usually go to their doctor and allow someone else to make all the decisions for them. Of course, they suffer a lot and finally die after having no quality of life, although they did spend a lot of money on their own "medical suicide."

In my experience, no one has ever been cured by chemotherapy, radiation or surgery—ever! If someone survives the pharmaceutical poisoning and the medical attacks, they survive in spite of the terror attack on their life not because of it.

I believe the statistics that show that 1/3 of all patients diagnosed with cancer never had it in the first place and were false positives, treated with all the horrors of the medical cabinet. Most of them will never even know that their breast was cut off without a good reason, and that the massive damage done by the chemotherapy and radiation is also causing cancer and early death.

Just think about it: Chemotherapy is a leftover of the First and Second World Wars. It is based on the chemicals that were created for warfare to kill people on the battlefield. After the wars were over they had no idea what to do with all the chemical poisons they came up with, so the absurd idea was to put the dangerous Mustard Gas (after the Geneva Convention forbade it to be used as a war chemical) into humans. The basis of this completely ridiculous idea, one which wasn't founded on any good science, was to kill the human to a point where all cells and body functions are dead but the patient is still somewhat alive.

After this terrible near death experience only the good and healthy cells are supposed to re-grow and the cancer cells won't come back. Well, that would be the same as if you went into your garden and killed all the flowers, trees and grass together with some weeds, hoping that only the flowers, trees and grass would grow back, but not the weeds. The same happens with chemotherapy.

If you have ever seen someone going into the hospital with cancer he or she usually looks and acts pretty normal until they poison them a couple of times with what they call chemotherapy. The person then looks 10 or 15 years older within days or weeks. Not only does their hair fall out, but their fingernails, gums and teeth often start rotting away. The person is sterile and often impotent, and can no longer be an organ donor, even after just one chemotherapy session.

The quality of life is usually gone instantly and a slow death is spread out as long as possible to make as much money as they can on the poor patient. The wasting away problem that is usually the final cause of death for the medically treated cancer patient begins right away.

If the medical victim does not show any improvement, they move to radiation therapy. Radiation, as well as chemotherapy, causes cancer and does nothing except burn away the size of the mutation (tumor), builds scars and creates toxic deposits for the development of new cancerous growth. No one wants to live next to a nuclear reactor because they know that radiation causes cancer the same way an atomic bomb would do if you survived the major explosion.

Slaughter or, as they call it, *surgery*, knocks out the immune system first with the anesthesia and all of the implemented medication then destroys it even more with the massive physical trauma that comes with every surgery. This is usually the route the medical field takes in cases of fast spreading or fast growing cancer.

More cancers are caused by the so-called early detection methods which were really created as a way to generate more customers. The medically treated patient usually dies anyway at a given time, but the earlier they detect the cancer the longer they are able to make money on the patient because they can treat him longer.

Isn't it strange that the cancer patient usually gets the most amounts of chemotherapy in the last days of their life? Is it just me or does this very clearly show that they're trying to make every dime they can on the poor victim before he or she is finally gone?

Oh yes, and then after they have tried every murderous approach on their victim and the patient hasn't gotten any better, there are always new and untested drugs or treatments, and they finish off the patient with the rest of that stuff.

As you can see, I don't believe that the medical profession has any acceptable approach to cancer and they should just stay out of it, especially since they have taken the Hippocratic Oath: First, do no harm!

It is not really the medical doctor—even if they are the main cause of death in America—that should bear all of the fault because it is truly their limited education and the manipulation and brainwashing created by the pharmaceutical industry that is causing these damaging and saddening results. The big pharmaceutical industry bribes its way into all kinds of powerful positions and is able to influence and make laws assuring that no natural cancer cure will ever be legally implemented in America or Europe. As we all know by now…it's all about the money.

You Don't Have To Die Of Cancer

The true number one cause of death in the Western world is the US government or, better said, their criminal institutions like the FTC, FDA and all of the others. Since the new CEO of the United States of America Incorporated, Barack Obama, does not even try to hide in whose interest he works, it is more dangerous than ever before. He makes sure that he moves as quickly as possible before anyone finds out what he's really doing.

The laws and regulations Obama makes, or allows to be made, are in favor of the pharmaceutical and medical industry, as well as for genetically manipulated food GMO which could potentially make you infertile, impotent and sick, and then finally kill you because we don't have the enzymes to deal with it. Plus, the murderous techniques that are allowed to produce this junk food will cause a completely new form of disease.

That's How They Give Us Cancer

It's not enough that the government gives us cancer by radiating our food, allowing thousands of chemicals to be put into our food, and by putting fluoride and chlorine and drugs into our drinking water, but they also vaccinate us—which is the main cause for all deadly forms of disease.

Diseases like cancer, Parkinson's, Alzheimer's, Multiple Sclerosis, Muscular Dystrophy, autism, sudden infant death syndrome, brain tumors and so on are all caused by inoculations. Vaccination is an assault with a deadly weapon and has never been proven safe and effective. In countries that do not vaccinate against polio and small pox the infections disappeared much faster than vaccinating countries. The reason is better nutrition and hygiene, not vaccinations.

Vaccines contain so many toxins that it is easy to understand why people get so sick and die from them. You can read about it in my book *Instinct Based Medicine How to Survive Your Illness and Your Doctor.*

Case Study of Healing with IBMS™
Recovery from Bone Cancer

When Hans came to my office, he was in pitiful shape. He used to be an accomplished athlete and worked professionally as a building engineer. Now he was unable to climb stairs and could hardly move. Hans spent his days in a wheelchair or in bed, as he suffered from severe pain. The doctor diagnosed Hans with Spinal Muscular Atrophy.

Even though Hans was stricken with illness, I was impressed by his courage. He said, "As long as I can breathe, I will fight." As we began to talk, I discovered that Hans wanted nothing less than optimum health. We began by stimulating his brain because the healing and regeneration process is initiated by the brain.

Doctors had given Hans a maximum life expectancy of 12 to 18 months. Although they offered no hope for healing or recovery, Hans courageously placed himself in my care for IBMS™ self-healing and therapy.

I asked Hans to visualize himself at a fitness center, which was filled with symbols that facilitated healing. Because the subconscious works with symbols, Hans worked out step-by-step in his mind. He visualized himself using a variety of exercise equipment. With each mental workout, Hans strengthened every single muscle in his body. He programmed his conscious to see himself as healthy and strong. He visualized himself interacting with his children and wife as a healthy man. These mental exercises strongly motivated Hans, and enabled his subconscious to perform the powerful act of healing from this incurable illness. After four weeks, Hans was completely pain free. Ultimately, Hans activated his self-healing power and created a new quality of life for himself.

Today, Hans is one of my best friends. Whenever I see him, he is happy and filled with zest for life. I share his story because it confirms that everyone possesses a God-given power to heal himself. Dear reader, you too can improve the quality of your life, even if you are severely ill, if you are willing to do whatever is necessary to restore your health.

THE "DR. COLDWELL PROTOCOL™"

Here is the Historical Protocol used by Dr. Coldwell for his patients, and that is used by the MDs and NDs and NMD s that have been personally trained and licensed by Dr. Leonard Coldwell. (This is of course for educational and research purposes only because many political, medical and financial powers don't want you to use this success proven and effective protocol.) Let me tell you at this point: "I do not practice Medicine I do practice HEALTH!"

The "Dr. Coldwell Protocol™"

I am convinced that the only cause of cancer, with the exception of accidents or assaults like radiation, poison or physical trauma of all kind, is Stress! Mainly mental and emotional stress!

The absolute only way to get and stay healthy is to define and eliminate the root cause of your individual health challenge with your individual " Only Answer!" And here is how my patients defined and learned how to eliminate the root cause of their personal health challenges and how to eliminate this root cause of their individual conflicts! If you eliminate the root cause that lead to your individual health challenge and eliminate this specific root cause with your personal individual "Only Answer" the symptoms (illness, disease and conditions) will disappear on their own, if you give your body the physical foundation to be healthy!

Defining the root cause of your individual health challenge:
Therefore the first questions I asked each of my patients was: (please write your answers down)

1. **What is it that made sick?**

   I know many of you think you don't know the answer, but if I insist that you write something down – what would your answer be?

   - Trauma from the past that you cannot let go of?

   - A bad relationship in the present or past?

   - Your job?

   - Where in your life do you make constant compromises against yourself – against your true personality or what you truly desire or stand for?

   - Which fears, worries and doubts are nagging on you that are creating chronic stress in your life?

     So answer me my dear friend – truly what is it that makes you sick?

2. **Where are your personal challenges with yourself?**

   - Do you love yourself?

   - Do you have self confidence and self esteem and a sense of self worthiness?

   - If not, and here it comes: WHY NOT?

3. **Where are you going?**

   - Do you have clear goals?

   - Motivation?

   - A reason for living?

- Something that makes you excited about yourself and your life and future?

- What do you want to have, be or achieve in the next 5 years? 10 years? 50 years? Remember, goals give you motivation to act!

4. **Who are the energy drainers in your life that need to go?:**

I mean the people that are always negative – that make you feel bad about yourself, your life, your goals and dreams and that make you feel weak or drained whenever you have do deal with them in person, on the phone or any situation? Make a list and eliminate them from your life! – Very often the root cause of cancer is simply a bad relationship. If you are married to the wrong person – get out of the marriage and start a new relationship ASAP!

You can easily find answers to all the speed bumps that you define by answering the questions above honestly and truthfully or you can use my CD set: Healing Life™ to do that! You find all the information on my educational self help sessions on www.instinctbasedmedicine.com and you should also listen to my archived and new radio shows to get more valuable information! Simply go to: http://www.blogtalkradio.com/search/Dr.-leonard-coldwell/archives and read my Daily Blog on: http://thedrcoldwellreport.blogspot.com

The physical causes:
As we all know by now the chemicals in our diet can kill us. Therefore it is more than important to eliminate all environmental toxins and the chemicals in our food as much as we can and to detoxify the body systemically and regularly!

1. **Stay away from Aspartame** and all artificial sweeteners and also know that even stevia, due to the process of making it, can be highly toxic. I use only *Just Like Sugar* from www.justlikesugarinc.com. For

information on this product see my good friend Dr. Betty Martini's website www.dorway.com. Stay away from high fructose corn syrup and any other form of artificial sweetener – whatsoever!

2. **Eat organic** as much as you can afford and support your body with the best living and life giving nutrients along with safe and effective supplements (because there are not enough nutrients in the food any longer). I use quint essence, vitamin e, d and flora zymes from www.awesomesupplements.com every day. I only use their products and individual cleanses for reasons of safety and effectiveness.

3. **The importance of hydration** is tremendous! Dehydration is the main physical cause of premature aging, illness and death. My patients drink at least a gallon of living energy rich water (please get informed about living water and safe filtration: www.ewater.com). Our body is built mainly from water that needs to be refreshed on a regular basis or it will become a rotten body of water, like a river that stops flowing and does not get new fresh water from the well. In about 3 days the river will be toxic and all life in it will disappear – so will your body if you don't renew and refresh it all the time!

4. **Oxygen!** We can live 6 weeks without food, 6 days without water, but not even 6 minutes without oxygen! Oxygen is the main physical healer, but also our main source of energy! Start to breathe deep into your stomach to supply your body with oxygen and drink a lot of freshly made green juices. Everything green gives you chlorophyll and therefore oxygen into your body and it helps you also to get or keep your body alkaline! Some physical activity in fresh air and sun will also help you with that as well as oxygen therapy, and the expert controlled use of 35% food grade hydrogen peroxide! For more information please visit www.instinctbasedmedicine.com

5. **Detoxification:** since we are bombarded by toxins when breath, drink and eat, we need to detoxify our body on a regular basis. Since

most cleanses I know are highly toxic, worthless or unpredictable, I created, together with my MD colleagues, a cleansing protocol that cleanses the entire body on a cellular level in just 21 days, and helps the body eliminate acidosis and toxemia, which are the foundation or main physical cause of all illness and infections like the flu or cancer, as Noble Price winners Otto Warburg and Max Plank have scientifically proven. The only individual cleanses I have used with my patients on top of the foundational BePureCleansingSystem™ (see the information on www.mybepure.com. I do the cleanse system twice a year) is the Candida and Parasite Cleanse from www.awesomesupplements.com and the metal cleanse and test kit for metal toxification from www.helpingamericanow.com. Also a juicing fast or cleanse is wonderful, but can have some major side effects if you don't have close access to a restroom.

6. **Chronic Inflammation** is the most dangerous condition for health, energy and youthfulness! Historically, I use Hydrosol Silver from www.helpingamericanow.com and the Vitamin D 3 (up to 3 times 50,000 IU a day in extreme cases and 15,000 on a daily basis) and vitamin C and E as well as flora zymes and universal greens from www.awesomesupplements.com to conquer inflammation. You have to make sure, if you want to be in the best state of health that you can, to eliminate naturally all chronic inflammation, Candida overgrowth, toxemia, acidosis, lack of oxygen and dehydration. This elimination is simple and easy if you use the techniques and products mentioned in this book.

7. **Drugs!** The number one cause of disease, and most of all new diseases and conditions, are the effects of drugs, prescription and over the counter. If it is not a matter of life and death in an emergency situation, I would never take any drugs into my system.

8. **Don't be a fanatic!** Quality of life is very important for your health and you should enjoy life to the fullest. I found that if you do 70%

right you can do 30% wrong without major danger if you listen to your instincts and use common sense. But if you are sick, you have to do 100% of the right thing.

9. **Stress reduction, sleep and regeneration:** Stress, in my opinion, is the only cause of illness, depression, anxiety, early aging and death! Stress leads to dehydration, nutritional deficiencies, heart attacks, strokes, cancer and all other mental, emotional and physical challenges. You can only heal or regenerate in a state of deep restful sleep! Therefore I created the IBMS™ State of Self conditioning in which your body is totally relaxed and your mind more alert and clear than ever before. (You cannot learn this from a book. YOU have to use my educational self help CD's or licensed IBMS Coach™ to learn how to get, in 20 minutes, the benefits of 7 to 8 hours of deep restful sleep (according to the Berlin Health Institute and a major study that was conducted to test the effectiveness of the Dr. Coldwell System™) I created, to my knowledge, the only self programming and self conditioning and educational self help system that can enable you to eliminate all past and present trauma that may cause mental and emotional stress (this stress makes you or keeps you away from perfect health) and lets you recondition your own programming for your happiness, life, success and wellness in just 20 minutes.

10. **The neurological conditioning of optimum health and healing!** Since the brain has no way of telling the difference between a real event or an imagined one you can live or relive everything in your mind, and program, delete or reprogram everything you want. We are all built out of atoms which means pure energy, and energy does not need time to change. If you switch on a lamp the light comes on. In the same way you can change your body, your mind and emotional existence and reality in seconds. That explains spontaneous healing which I have witnessed and produced in my life very often. Tumors the size of a fist can disappear in seconds.

The main elements in the effective self programming sessions are first: to acknowledge the fact that something is wrong. Positive thinking " I am healthy – I am healthy" or to simply ignore the problem will definitely kill you or at least will prevent healing! You have to accept the challenge, and tell the body what is wrong and how to deal with the health challenge to activate all of your self healing powers. Then focus on the tumor for example (like in my audio session: Self Healing) and imagine light or healing warmth or whatever feels right to you penetrating the tumor and these forces are eliminating the tumor. See it shrinking and disappearing and at the end see yourself in a state of total health, happiness and wellbeing to give your body and nervous system the goal and reason and end result you want to achieve.

You can also imagine that you forgive someone the hurt you in the past and set them and yourself free of their negative emotional influence on your life and health as well as even tell someone in the IBMS State™ all the things good or bad, calm or angry what you always wanted to tell them and repeat it until it has no negative emotional or physical influence on your body and life anymore. Then just let them go and never ever even think about them or the incident anymore.

It sounds very simple and easy and it actually is! Because in the IBMS state™, your body is totally relaxed and gives your brain all the energy that the body does not need in this relaxed state and gives you the clearest and strongest state of mind possible. Now in this state, using the music in my audio session, you can experience a total hemispheric synchronization that means that both sides of the brain can work at the same time, and this gives you more neurological resources to use your brain capacity then in any other state of mind. Since your thoughts are not filtered by doubts and fears or limitations from the conscious thinking rationalizing part of the brain, you can program, reprogram or condition your brain in any way you want to produce any result you want to achieve.

You can do a similar programming in any relaxed state when

your mind is sharp and clear, but it will take a dramatically longer timeframe to achieve similar results. You do this kind of programming since the day you are born anyway. It simply works by repetition too! So my CD's are not necessarily needed to achieve the results you try to achieve, they can simply enable you to produce faster results much easier.

You always start by acknowledging the problem and show your brain what you want to happen and what the end result should be. That stimulates your neurology to work on the realization of your programming.

11. **The stress reduction part** is in my opinion the most important and often the only part needed for a change in your well being. Simply define the situations and people that are causing stress in your life and create an action plan on how to eliminate the situation or people from your life or to deal with it more effectively. If someone calls you an Idiot, for example, you can react on it with aggression or depression or simply say: "you have an interesting opinion" and just let it go and not even touch you emotionally. It is not what happens that creates our emotional experiences in life it is how we react to it that makes all the difference in your life. Therefore, simply define the stressors in your life and work on action plans to eliminate them or at least their impact on your life and health. Use my book *Instinct Based Medicine: How to survive your Illness and your doctor*, www.instinctbasedmedicine.com to develop action plans or use books and CDs from great speakers and teachers like Zig Ziglar or Og Mandino or Earl Nightingale!

12. **The use of healing elements! (As usual for educational and research purposes only)** To speed up the physical recovery my doctors use the protocol I personally developed in all these years of research and success. The main protocol my doctors use with cancer patients is:

To create the foundation of detoxification and alkalinity it begins with the BePureCleansingSystem from www.mybepure.com and the metal cleanse at the same time from www.helpingamericanow.com and the use of Universal Greens from www.awesomesupplements. com and the instant implementation of intra Venous injection of 10 grams of vitamin C a day for 21 days (many doctors also use Aloe Vera IV injections) plus the use of Essiac Tea or I prefer Capsules from www.awesomesupplements.com and 3 times 50 000 IU of Vitamin D 3 from the same company for 21 days and after that 25 000 IU ones a day until they are perfectly fine. The maintenance doses is 15 000 IU a day for life.

All patients in Europe have to do 3 IMBS Audio Sessions™ a day (more if they like). All of my patients always had to go on a total raw food diet as you find at www.paulnison.com and at the end of this book as well as the information from all the great raw foodists at the end of my book. The juicing detoxification starts with apple, celery and carrot juice mixed 1/3rd each in the morning on an empty stomach and continued with at least 4 large glasses of fresh organic juices a day. Get Jack Lalanes books and his juicer, if you like, for more information about juicing.

All patients in the European IBMS Centers™ are given at least a gallon of water filtered by filters and vitalized by products from my dear friend Fred Van Liew from www.ewater.com and all get his Electro Magnetic Frequency protectors to be safe from all the damaging and cancer causing micro waves from computers, cell phones and so on. We even use a specific Pendant during the IBMS Sessions™ to help the patient to relax faster and easier.

We also use Oxygen Multi Step Therapy after Prof. Manfred von Ardenne and up to 25 drops of 35% food grade Hydrogen Peroxide in 8 ounces of aloe juice 3 times a day. But you cannot just do it or take it before you have educated yourself, and or are supervised by someone that can legally help you with this H2O2 protocol, because used in the wrong way it can be highly toxic and damaging to your health and life. Often the medical director of my centers used DMSO and Cesium injections, as well as other elements mentioned in the book, if he felt it was the right thing to do. My colleague Dr. Crone MD ND HD often use a nebulizer if patients did not want or like injections to get the healing elements he decided on into the bloodstream of his patients.

We always add Laetrile or Vitamin B 17.

The daily supplementation we use after the 21 days of cleansing is quint essence, vitamin e, c and d as well as Essiac capsules or tea and good bio available calcium.

As I mentioned before there are over 300 known safe and effective natural cures available in nature to eliminate the symptoms (tumors, mutated cells and every other form of unnatural growth or mutation), but that does not cure cancer. These natural cures only help the body to eliminate the symptoms of cancer.

Cancer is a disease of the mind, if not caused by toxins, assaults and accidents, or by chemotherapy and radiation, or spread fast and aggressively because of surgery. The only way to be cancer free is to define and eliminate the root cause of cancer. If you find and eliminate the root cause of your individual lack of energy that make cancer or all other disease possible in the first place then all health challenges will disappear on their own with common sense help of living hydration and nutrition and detoxification and supplementation.

Now you have the Only Answer! And the only answer to cancer for you can only be the single one individual answer you will find for yourself out of trial and error and the use of the information I give you in this book and my books *Instinct Based Medicine, The Only Answer to Stress, Anxiety and Depression* and *You are born to win*. Research, learn, try and make educated decisions and take action. Don't put your health and life into the hands of someone else, at least not without doing your own research first and if you have any further question go to www.instinctbasedmedicine.com. This website will be constantly updated or simply write me an email to instinctbasedmedicine@gmail.com, but not if I have to answer spam filters like from eathlink etc I simply don't have the time and will not bother to fill them out.

The Only Answer to Cancer – to your individual Cancer – can only be your personal individual Answer to your individual cancer. You created your personal health challenges knowingly or unknowingly and you are the only one that has the power and tools to eliminate them. Remember:" There is no healing force outside the human body" if you don't do it nobody can. And if you decide to go the medical route you should do it full heartedly because whatever you decide on do it 100%. Doubt will just kill you. And, as I stated already, all patients I ever saw that did both the alternative and medical treatments together – died.

At the end it is your decision your life and your health and you are the only person that has to live with the consequences of your decisions and actions, and not me or the MD that you may follow for treatment. So use education, common sense and most of all your instinct and I am sure you will make the right decision!

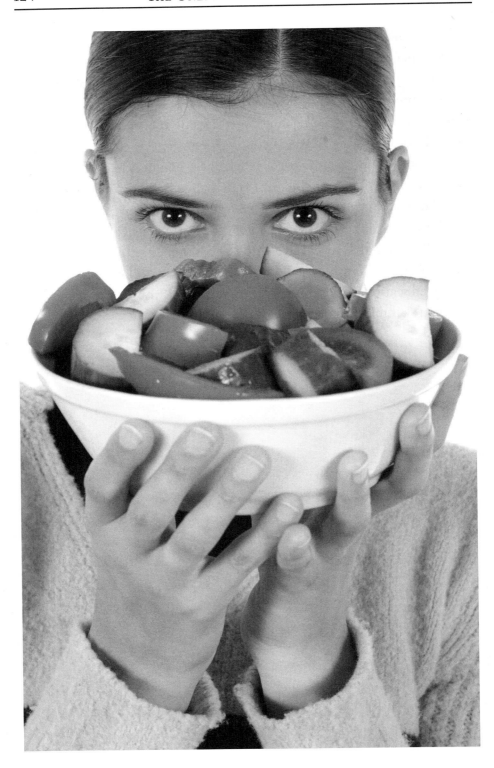

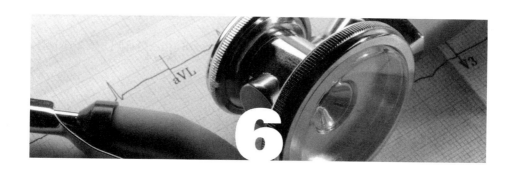

WAYS TO PREVENT CANCER FROM COMING BACK

It's important to keep your liver, gallbladder, and kidneys working efficiently. You can do that by flushing them once or more a year. With the Be Pure Cleansing system from www.MyBePure.com and by doing every 6 months the metal cleanse from www.HelpingAmericanow.com and by doing the Candida and Parasite cleanse from www.Awesome-Supplements.com once a year too.

German physicians and scientists pioneered enzyme therapy, which all of the German cancer clinics recommend. Enzyme therapy can help prevent cancer from coming back. To get more enzymes, increase your intake of raw fruits and vegetables. You can also get enzyme supplements from www.AwesomeSupplements.com. Also, my family and I take their Quint-Essence, Flora-Zymes, vitamin E, D and C, every day of our lives.

Once a year we do a 3 week organic whole food diet from www.GreatWholeFood.com and take only their safe toothpaste, deodorant and soaps.

But at the end of the day I believe it is the applied IBMS™ sessions that they use daily that keeps them healthy.

You Can't Pick And Choose Just One Thing

I am always stunned that some people want to cure a life threatening disease or condition that took decades to create with just one single, cheap supplement or herb. This simply will not work! If you're facing a health challenge, it did not happen over night. In fact, it took many years and tens of thousands of dollars along with a lot of bad choices to make yourself sick. There's no way you can take a single pill and heal from these massive, life threatening health break downs.

You can't eat junk foods and pour toxins into your body for ten, twenty, thirty or more years then just swallow a multi-vitamin or the "newest cure" and be healthy and full of energy within a week.

Thyroid problems, diabetes and high blood pressure are more prevalent now than ever. However, it's not due to genetic problems, it's due to overeating, bad choices, and an unhealthy lifestyle in general. Let's face it, you're overweight and will die much earlier than you should. But the good news is you don't have to *stay* overweight! No, it's not easy to make changes in your life, but it's absolutely necessary if you want to live a healthy, happy, successful life.

I have seen the illnesses and symptoms that are caused by obesity. It's killing you! All of the fat on your body is accumulated toxins and poisons that the body stores in your fat cells, the more overweight you are, the more toxic your body is.

In many ways I believe in tough love. I always hit my patients hard— mentally and emotionally. Why? Because so many people are under a sort of self-hypnosis and I try to snap them out of it! Only when you wake up will you be able to change. If you are willing to accept that you created your high blood pressure, diabetes 2, cancer, or any other health problem and are willing to reverse the bad choices that got you here, I will do everything in my power to educate, coach, support and help you on your way to optimal health.

However, if you're looking for a magic pill or a miracle cure that will fix all of your problems without you taking charge and control over your own life and health, then this book is not for you. Since you're still reading though, I can tell that you're a determined person, eager to make sweeping life changes both inside and out.

Do you swat mosquitoes or drain the swamp?

The typical American cancer doctor focuses on the cancer and is looking for a way to get rid of them instead of stabilizing the patient so that his body can do the work to get rid of the cancer cells. But he makes up his mind to get rid of those cancer cells one way or another—"whatever it takes."

Usually step one is to cut the cancerous growth out of the body. And so if the cancer is operable, the tumor is surgically removed. But everyone today knows that even the medical profession knows that if a few cancer cells are left behind in the body after surgery they will start new cancerous growth. And in the approach to kill off those cells, step two is to burn the cancer cells out of the body by radiation—which causes cancer, toxic scar tissue, etc.

And just to make *triple* sure all those cancer cells are gone, step three is to poison any remaining cancer cells with chemotherapy—which also causes cancer.

The problem is, cancer usually returns because nobody tried to even approach, identify and eliminate the root cause of the patient's cancer which is always related to mental and emotional stress. Instead, they treat cancer as if it's a localized and not a systemic phenomenon.

Remember, I believe cancer does not exist as an illness, it is an accumulation of symptoms that are based on negative frequency's, or, better said, being out of homeostasis —being out of balance.

It is always lack of energy that leads to cancer! And if this lack of energy does not get eliminated will the patient die? Without a doubt! And all along the "cancer cure route" what happens if the patient doesn't heal? More surgery? More radiation? More chemo? When cancer patients have received their lifetime quota of radiation, they can't have any more of it—even if the cancer returns.

The most chemotherapy is usually given the last weeks of a cancer patients life to make as much money as possible before the "customer is gone." As for chemo, it's toxic and kills healthy cells. Worst of all, it often has no effect on the tumors at all. The tumors keep growing as if there's no tomorrow, despite massive doses of the most toxic chemotherapies known to man. It's almost as if some cancers thrive on chemo. That is because chemo does cause new cancer growth plus it weakens the immune system so much that the body cannot fight the cancer cell multiplication any more on its own.

Sadly, the American approach to cancer treatment ("cut-burn-poison") is all too often a dead end. In other cases it leaves cancer patients disfigured from surgery or sickened or weakened.

If one may compare the cancer cell to another pesky parasite, the mosquito, the American-style cancer treatments are like swatting mosquitoes while ignoring the mosquitoes' breeding ground: the swamp. And that's why it often fails. Swatting mosquitoes isn't enough. It's necessary to drain the swamp!

Whether you receive conventional cancer treatment, alternative treatment, or a combination, if you want to get rid of cancer *for good* so that it *never* returns, you have to get serious about draining the swamp.

The German cancer specialists recognize that cancer is never a localized problem. In other words, breast cancer isn't simply a disease of the breast, and prostate cancer isn't simply a disease of the prostate. Rather, cancer is a symptom of a systemic disease of the *whole body*—no matter where the tumor may appear.

Plus, it's not physical anyway it is an energetic problem.

Something within the body is producing the cancer cells. When people get cancer, it means that their bodies have become the "swamp" (the breeding ground—mentally and emotionally and that causes the physical acidosis and toxemia) that allows the "mosquitoes" (cancer cells) to breed, multiply, and spread out of control.

It's necessary to clean up the body's toxic mess—in your mind and in your body.

It is a fact that a cancer patient's body is loaded with toxic wastes and toxic metals. Typically, a cancer patient's colon is junked up, his blood is thick and sludge-like, his lymphatic system is stagnant, his liver is clogged, his gall bladder accumulates stones, his kidneys are weak, and so on.

Because the cancer patient's organs are usually functioning inefficiently, toxins come into the body faster than the patient can get rid of them. That has to be reversed. And it can be!

"Draining the swamp" involves a serious detoxification process. A three-week course of treatment at a German cancer clinic can give you a good start at detoxification, but it's *only* a start. You have to continue the detoxification at home. It's an ongoing lifelong project. That is why I only endorse the 21 day full body and colon cleansing system from www.MyBePure.com. That is the world's only scientific system that I know of that will cleanse the body on a cellular level and it needs to be, for scientific reasons, a 21 day program.

The Be Pure Cleansing system is gentle but consistent and fast at the same time because usually the cancer patients I saw had only weeks or a month left to live—if you could believe their doctors. Because of this, I did not have time to cleanse them organ by organ for 9 months.

Cleanse the colon

The German doctors recognize the necessity of "draining the swamp." That's why they *all* recommended colonic hydrotherapy to their patients—a low-tech treatment most orthodox doctors ignore or even discourage. The colon is the center of the "swamp." You can easily do colonic hydrotherapy in the privacy of your home, unless you prefer to pay for the services of a professional colonic hydro therapist.

Change your body from acidic to alkaline

An acidic body is the foundation for cancer, and cancer cells thrive in an acidic oxygen lacking environment. The typical average diet, which is high in meat, high in sugar, and low in fruits and vegetables, contributes to an acidic body.

To change from an acidic body to an alkaline body, you can't eat like the typical American. You must eliminate refined sugar because cancer cells love sugar. If you're fighting cancer, stop feeding it! Cut the cancer cells off from their favorite food: sugar. Switch from a high meat diet to one that has little or no meat. Especially avoid red meat.

Eat lots of fruits and vegetables—organic if possible. A fresh lemonade morning tonic, which you can use to start your day, can help change your body from acidic to alkaline.

Here's the recipe for lemonade:

Squeeze the juice out of a lemon and add two tablespoons of *authentic* Grade B maple syrup—or an amount that suits your taste. You can use Grade A maple syrup, but don't use any kind of cheap, sugary, artificial maple syrup. Add about 10 to 12 ounces of water and some ground cayenne pepper, and stir well or shake it in a shaker cup. You can start with a pinch of cayenne and gradually work your way up to a half-teaspoon. According to some doctors this lemonade has other benefits, too. It digests mucus, increases circulation, and stimulates the body to produce the hydrochloric acid necessary for digestion.

I love my special lemonade: 3 apples and ¼ of a lemon with peel—organic, clean and ice cold! Try it.

Flush your lymphatic system

If there are too many toxins in your body they get stuck in your lymphatic system. As discussed before, unlike your circulatory system, your lymphatic system doesn't have a pump, and we have 4 times more lymph liquid in our body then blood.

There are only two ways to flush your lymphatic system: through aerobic exercise such as swimming or biking, or lymphatic drainage massage which is 1000% more effective and faster and can make sure nothing toxic is left in the lymph nodes.

Help your largest organ—your skin—eliminate waste and renew itself

Sweating is good because it helps your body get rid of toxins through your skin, which is your body's largest organ. Taking a hot sauna and finishing it with a cold shower helps to do this. But an even more effective sauna is the far infrared sauna, which quickly and easily pulls out toxins from deep within the skin. This kind of sauna can even be installed in your home.

Another technique for assisting your skin is dry skin brushing: using no water, you brush every square inch of your skin with a natural bristle brush every day. Why? There are several benefits: it cleans pores, exfoliates the skin, keeps skin toned and soft, AIDS, blood circulation, and helps eliminate toxins. Dry skin brushing also stimulates all of your body's acupuncture points, which helps energize the body.

Read what the legendary natural healer Dr. Bernard Jensen said about dry skin brushing: "I believe skin brushing is one of the finest of all baths. No soap can wash the skin as clean as the new skin you have under the old. You make new skin every 24 hours on the body. The skin will be as clean as the blood is. Skin brushing removes the top layer. This helps to eliminate uric acid crystals, catarrh, and various other acids in the body. The skin should eliminate two pounds of waste acids daily. Keep the skin active."

You'll need two different brushes for dry skin brushing: a body brush with a removable handle and a complexion brush.

Get rid of the false, negative programming in your mind to eliminate cancer.

An often overlooked part of the "swamp" is the mind, and that is my most favorite playing and battle field. All illness is in the mind before it is manifested in the body. Therefore, all health is in the mind before you can experience it in the body. It's necessary to detoxify the mind! By getting rid of the false, negative thoughts, worries, doubts and fears as well as lack of motivation, low self-esteem, lack of self-love, hopelessness and the feeling of being helpless, you can get rid of cancer.

Toxic thinking should be replaced with healing thoughts that kick your immune system into high gear. Most of the German clinics help the patient focus on this very task, and this is something you can also do at home. Believe it or not, counseling techniques that change the cancer patient's thought patterns have turned around "hopeless" and "terminal" cases of cancer.

It's not just a matter of changing from "negative thinking" to "positive thinking"—though that's part of it. More importantly, it's a matter of changing *false* thinking to *true* thinking. For example, many if not most cancer patients believe cancer is a powerful, almost invincible enemy. But the American pioneer O. Carl Simonton, M.D., points out that the truth is quite different: *cancer cells are, in fact, weak, abnormal, and deformed.* Dr. Simonton created a groundbreaking method that helps cancer patients visualize their immune system vanquishing the weak, deformed cancer cells.

Please read Dr. Bernie Siegel's books. He offers hope, inspiration and guidance to so many.

But the fastest and most effective way to achieve these necessary changes is, in my experience and the opinion of thousands of my patients and colleagues, the IBMS™. It does not allow space for failure.

The Effects of Chemotherapy

A
Abdominal Pain
Acid Indigestion
Acid Reflux
Allergic Reactions
Alopecia
Anaphylaxis
Anemia
Anxiety
Appetite (Lack Of)
Arthralgias
Asthenia
Ataxia
Azotemia

B
Balance & Mobility Changes

Bilirubin Blood Level
Bone Pain
Bladder Problems
Bleeding Problems
Blood Clots
Blood Pressure Changes
Blood Test Abnormalities
Breathing Problems
Bronchitis
Bruising

C
Cardiotoxicity
Cardiovascular Events
Cataracts
Central Neurotoxicity
Chemo Brain

Chest Pain
Chills
Cognitive Problems
Cold Symptoms
Confusion
Conjunctivitis (Pink Eye)
Constipation
Cough
Cramping
Cystitis

D
Deep Vein Thrombosis (DVT)
Dehydration
Depression
Diarrhea
Dizziness
Drug Reactions
Dry Eye Syndrome
Dry Mouth
Dry Skin
Dyspepsia
Dyspnea

E
Early Satiety
Edema
Electrocardiogram (ECG/EKG)
Changes
Electrolyte Imbalance
Esophagitis
Eye Problems

F
Fatigue
Feeling Faint
Fertility
Fever
Flatulence
Flu-like Syndrome
Flushing

G
Gas
Gastric Reflux
Gastroesophageal Reflux Disease
(GERD)
Genital Pain

Granulocytopenia
Gynecomastia
Glaucoma

H
Hair Loss
Hand-Foot Syndrome
Headache
Hearing Loss
Hearing Problems
Heart Failure
Heart Palpitations
Heart Problems
Heart Rhythm Changes
Heartburn
Hematoma
Hemorrhagic Cystitis
Hepatotoxicity
High Blood Pressure (Hypertension)
High Liver Enzymes
Hyperamylasemia (High Amylase)
Hypercalcemia (High Calcium)
Hyperchloremia (High Chloride)
Hyperglycemia (High Blood Sugar)
Hyperkalemia (High Potassium)
Hyperlipasemia (High Lipase)
Hypermagnesemia (High Magnesium)
Hypernatremia (High Sodium)
Hyperphosphatemia (High Phosphate)
Hyperpigmentation
Hypersensitivity Skin Reactions
Hypertriglyceridemia (High
Triglycerides)
Hyperuricemia (High Uric Acid)
Hypoalbuminemia (Low Albumin)
Hypocalcemia (Low Calcium)
Hypochloremia (Low Chloride)
Hypoglycemia (Low Blood Sugar)
Hypokalemia (Low Potassium)
Hypomagnesemia (Low Magnesium)
Hyponatremia (Low Sodium)
Hypophosphatemia (Low Phosphate)

I
Impotence
Incoordination
Infection
Injection Site Reactions
Injury
Insomnia
Iron Deficiency Anemia
Itching

J
Joint Pain

K
Kidney Problems

L
Leukopenia
Liver Dysfunction
Liver Problems
Loss of Libido
Low Blood Counts
Low Blood Pressure
  (Hypotension)
Low Platelet Count
Low Red Blood Cell Count
Low White Blood Cell Count
Lung Problems

M
Memory Loss
Menopause
Metallic Taste
Mouth Sores
Mucositis
Muscle Pain
Myalgias
Myelosuppression
Myocarditis

N
Nail Changes
Nausea
Nephrotoxicity
Nervousness
Neutropenia
Neutropenic Fever
Nosebleeds
Numbness

O
Ototoxicity

P
Pain
Palmar-Plantar Erythrodysesthesia
Pancytopenia
Pericarditis
Peripheral Neuropathy
Pharyngitis
Photophobia
Photosensitivity
Pneumonia
Pneumonitis
Post-nasal Drip
Proteinuria
Pulmonary Embolus (PE)
Pulmonary Fibrosis
Pulmonary Toxicity

R
Radiation Recall
Rash
Rapid Heart Beat
Rectal Bleeding
Restlessness
Rhinitis
Ringing Ears
Runny Nose

S
Sadness
Seizures
Sexuality
Shortness of Breath
Sinusitis
Skin Reactions
Sleep Problems
Sore Mouth
Stomach Sour
Stomach Upset
Stomatitis
Swelling

T
Taste Changes
Thrombocytopenia
Thyroid Hormone Levels
Tingling
Tinnitus
Trouble Sleeping

U
Urinary Tract Infection

V
Vaginal Bleeding
Vaginal Dryness
Vaginal Infection
Vertigo
Vomiting

W
Water Retention
Watery Eyes
Weakness
Weight Changes
Weight Gain
Weight Loss

X
Xerostomia

Positive thinking alone does not work for Cancer patients!

The philosophy behind positive thinking is beneficial, but it does not work for Cancer patients. You can only heal yourself if you can imagine yourself healthy, vital and full of energy!

If you want to be as happy, healthy and successful as you can be, you have to do these things (The Law of Attraction and Attitude in Action):

- Program it into your conscious and subconscious through introspection

- Have a clear vision—precise goals

- Develop a detailed action plan for heatlh and healing (Which Therapies, Diet or Programs you want to use).

- Put your plan into action every single day to achieve and keep optimum health. (Keep your focus on the goal—optimum health—and use the Law of attraction.)

- Keep in mind that a lack of action is the beginning of death and decay! Your body needs active care. You cannot just think about a healthy diet and not doing it.

Listen to Kevin Trudeau's CD set: *Your wish is Your Command* to understand the difference between wishful thinking and really using the law of attraction. www.Ktradionetwork.com

As Dr. Bernie Siegel MD and Yale professor stated and I paraphrase, cancer patients that are positive thinking about their health situation and, for example, say: "I am healthy, I am fine" etc., give their immune system this information: "everything is fine—no reason to act—nothing to do!" Consequently, the cancer patient dies because he did not activate his immune system.

He shut it off instead of doing it IBMS™ technically right and saying: "I am severely ill! I accept this fact and activate now my self healing system and instincts, and I will act accordingly. Because I will do whatever it takes, and because I will follow my instincts and common sense and educate myself to make sophisticated decisions and put them into action I know I will be cured. I know that my body, mind and spirit knows how to heal me and I will do whatever it takes to be and stay healthy. And because I support my immune system and stimulate healing in myself, I know I will be healed. I am strong and getting stronger and healthier day by day, hour by hour, minute by minute and second by second. I know because I do all the rights things that my research and instinct is telling me: I will be happy and healthy very soon! I am on my way and I am excited because I know I am in complete control."

The IBMS™ CDs

I invested thousands of dollars finding the right music for the background of my CDs. This is important because the IBMS™ sessions are capable of scientifically changing your subconscious since it gets the listener into the right brain wave frequencies that are necessary to make changes. These CDs actually get you into the mental mode of living and experiencing your ideal life—which is the only way to successfully reprogram your mind.

There is no other system known worldwide today that can do what my IBMS™ does each and every time by getting your brain into the right frequencies of beta, alpha, delta and theta. This is very important and necessary for the right programming.

In the opinion of many leading healers, practitioners and successful MDs, there is no program out there that can produce even 1% of what the IBMS™ does and without any major effort on the part of the user. This program will help you to find solutions, create goals, develop an action plans and uncover the root cause of all life's challenges including health challenges and breakdowns of all kind.

The Berlin health institute has clinically proven that the IBMS™ equals the relaxation, regenerating and healing of 7 to 8 hours of deep restful sleep, just in one 20 minutes session! When you remember that the body can only heal while you are in a deep restful sleep or IBMS-State™ you will easily understand why it was so effective for my cancer and other patients.

My stress reduction system on CD is also available specifically for Christians and is called Quiet Time.

With the publication of this book I will, for the very first time ever, make my entire IBMS-Life Therapy System™ available for the public. Until now it was only available for the 143 MDs and PhDs that I trained as IBMS-Practitioners™ or IBMS Therapists™. Also, the IBMS™ seminars and courses for healers and practitioners will start with the publication of this book. We will also offer a special CD set for Cancer patients! For more information go to: www.InstinctBasedMedicine.com or write to InstinctBasedMedicine@gmail.com

The All Natural Approach

IBMS™ is the way nature intended you to stay healthy and to heal and repair yourself. It's the best way to prevent disease, and best of all it's a simple and effective treatment to rid the body of malignant, viral, bacterial and allergic disease by using the laws of nature to heal and by eliminating the root cause of all disease which is a lack of energy. As we talked about before, this lack of energy is mainly caused by mental and emotional stress and the health destroying behavior that often is the result from these stressors.

The medical profession loses nearly 100% of their patients within 5 years of the first diagnoses. Their method of "curing patients" annoys me so badly! They believe that their form of treatment is the only way to even attempt to cure cancer, and yet they have a dismal survival rate.

Natural methods are the answer. You need oxygen therapy in one form or the other, but even this is not a cure. You need an organic raw food diet, but this is not the cure. You need a lot of water and proper nutrition, but it is not the cure. No one thing is the cure for everything. All these things help to relieve the symptoms of your personal health breakdown, and they do help to speed up the healing process, but until you get rid of the root cause or your own health problems, you will never heal!

Again, think about the answer to these questions: What is it that made, and is making you, sick? What are the constant worries doubts and fears and compromises against yourself? Is it lack of self-esteem, self-love, self-confidence that drain your energy to the point that you developed these symptoms and created this energy breakdown?

Once you answer that question and act upon it you will have your individual Only Answer to Cancer! You just need to add the necessary 14% of healthy behavior and you are on your way to optimum health, happiness and success.

Case Study of Healing with IBMS™
Healing of Breast Cancer

I clearly remember the first time that Elaine came to my office. She was in her mid-thirties and suffered from breast cancer. The doctors removed her right breast and treated her twice with chemotherapy. Elaine was in terrible shape. Her hair was falling out. She was frightened and emotionally devastated.

After a short consultation, I learned that Elaine suffered from depression and a gripping angst. Since her early childhood, she was not able to leave the house or sleep in the dark alone. Elaine's constant fears led to an inner resignation and a decreased will to live. As she became more and more depressed, her body began to self-destruct.

Elaine was on the brink of a nervous breakdown. In therapy, we started doing relaxation exercises, which helped her, calm down and internalize a peaceful mental state. Elaine quickly learned that our feelings and emotional outlook affect our perspective on life. The quality of our life depends on our perception and what we think about is what our future will hold.

If someone can't envision the future, then healing is impossible.

Before anything else, a person must believe that a bright future and optimum health is conceivable. As all religious books of the world state over and over again, that faith (or the power of belief) is the greatest force in human existence. In the final analysis, everything depends on whether you believe in your own success and healing.

With simple techniques and exercises, as I have described in my book The Unlimited Power of the Subconscious, we eliminated Elaine's fears. Like a beautiful flower, she began to blossom. As therapy continued, Elaine visualized her life integrated with her career and husband, who lovingly and enthusiastically stood by her side. Within a few weeks, Elaine was vibrant and full of energy. Previously, the doctors had given a life expectancy of six months. Now, she had every reason to live with passion.

Two years later, Elaine returned to the center with a large knot protruding from the scars of her former operation. She was terribly frightened, but felt hopeful because of her success two years earlier. I referred Elaine to the chief of surgery in a nearby hospital, who discovered something astonishing. The first operation was terribly botched. The cancer had been cut in two and half of it remained in Elaine's body. As any physician can confirm, this woman would have had less than three months to live because she carried a severe malignant tumor, the size of a walnut, in her body. This is the worst thing that can happen to a patient. The chief of the hospital had never seen anything like this, nor thought it possible. Half of the tumor was left in Elaine's body, but the tumor had isolated itself and had been pushed upward by the body's attempt to expel it.

Once the tumor was surgically removed, there was no need for chemotherapy. Elaine was told that she would never again be able to have children, but she quickly became pregnant. For this reason, Elaine remained under my care during pregnancy. The doctors told her that her baby would be sick, and possibly suffer from birth defects. After nine months, Elaine gave birth to a healthy child. There were no complications or difficulties during the birth. Elaine's beautiful little girl is now five years old. She is full of life, energy, health and vitality.

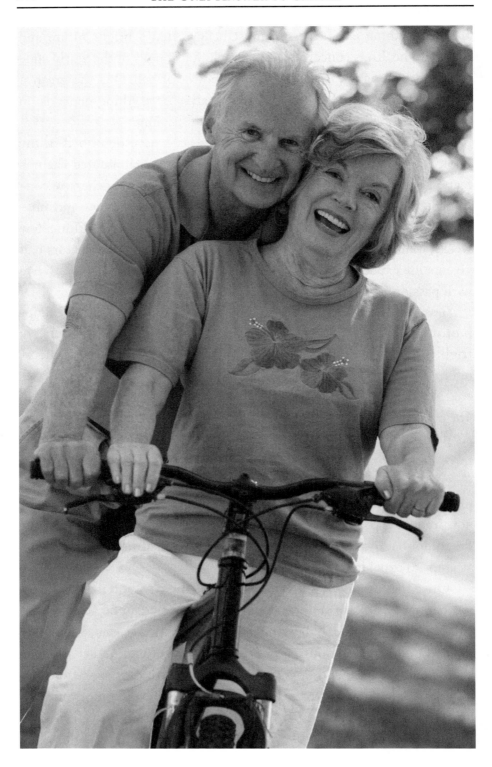

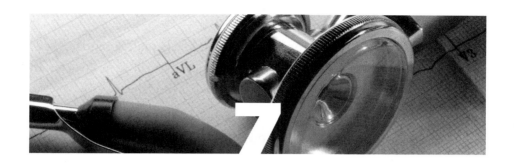

THE INSTINCT BASED MEDICINE SYSTEM™— IBMS™

We are now at the point where you should have a general understanding of the way I think, how I have cured cancer, and have helped many patients to cure themselves. If you have already read all of the facts and data in my book *Instinct Based Medicine: How to Survive Your Illness and Your Doctor*, you will understand that everything I've stated in this book is backed up by facts, experience and massive success.

If you are now ready to apply my IBMS™ into your life read on because I've put it all together for you.

The protocol for my IBMS™ as previously published in my books and papers is as follows:

1. Immediately go on a raw food diet. Become a vegetarian or vegan, at least until you are healthy again! I suggest using the Cancer Patient Diet from my friend Paul Nison in this book, but also read his other wonderful books or watch his video clips on Youtube:

    www.PaulNison.com

2. Stop drinking tap water, it's filled with poisons. Get a whole house water filter, or at the very least one that goes under sink. This should be a reverse osmosis system. Also put filters on all of your showers. You can get the best ones from: www.ewater.com

3. Avoid all artificial sweeteners like Aspartame, Equal, Splenda, Sweet n Low, and all others. Instead, use organic stevia as a sweetener. Never use MSG and stay away from GMO foods!

4. Don't consume milk or milk products such as yogurt, cheese and sour cream. Even milk in/or coffee is not allowed at this time.

5. Start juicing! The best and easiest to use is, in my opinion, the Jack Lalanne Juicer. You can get one at Cosco for a good price. Start every morning with a juice made from fresh apples, celery and carrot in equal proportions. Drink fresh juices at least four times a day. You can juice any fruits and vegetables you like, but remember that green vegetables give you oxygen and that is what cancer patients need most. You can go to my website for some juice recipes: www.InstinctBasedMedicine.com.

6. Drink a gallon of water every day with half a teaspoon of sea salt in it. Or, even better, use Stardust from www.GreatWholeFood.com You can also use their organic whole foods as snacks or as your general food.

7. Walk 28 minutes each day and expose your skin to the sun at least 12 minutes each day. Never use sunscreen because by now you know it could give you cancer.

8. Three times a day use a rebounder (mini-trampoline). Just bounce up and down without your feet leaving the fabric. Of course, a manual, full body lymph drainage on the parts of the body where the lymph knots are concentrated or painful and big, is best. However, some so-called medical professionals say this will spread the cancer into the entire system. I have had it done on all of my cancer patients and have never seen this happen!

9. Three times a day listen to the IBMS™ Stress Reduction CDs. (See info on www.InstinctBasedMedicine.com) And at least once a day you should use the Breathing Therapy session. When you've gotten used to this you can then switch over to the IBMS™ Immune and repair booster sessions.

10. Use the information in this book and/or my IBMS™ CD sessions: *Uncover and Eliminate the Root Cause.* This will help you to uncover the root cause of your individual energy and health break down. You'll be able to uncover the worries, fears, doubts that hold you back and are making you ill. You can also use my Self-Empowerment CD set and my book: *You are born to Win.* These are only suggestions. Everything you need to know is supplied in this book. Remember, all illness is the result of lack of energy. What is the root cause of your personal lack of energy? Find it and fix it, or you will not heal!

11. Now that hydration and nutrition have been covered, you need to start the detoxification process. I would start with the 21 day all-in-one full body and colon cleanse from www.MyBePure.com and after that the lymphatic, Candida and parasite cleanses from www.AwesomeSupplements.com I would take the metal cleanse and colloidal silver from www.HelpingAmericaNow.com and if you have the money take the Mega Bio Available Nutrition and super-hydration water from www.Trinisol.com.

12. The minimum requirement of supplementation is Essiac Capsules, one capsule of 400 IU vitamin E per 30 pounds of body weight, and 50, 000 IU vitamin D three times a day for the first week then lower the dose to 10,000 IU three times each day. Flaxseed oil is great for cancer, especially breast cancer. I would also take Quint-Essence, Tracite Liquid Fulvic Minerals and Flora-Zymes from www.AwesomeSupplements.com Also, see my full cancer protocol at www.InstinctBasedMedicine.com.

13. Only under the care of a qualified practitioner you can try:
    - Oxygen therapy after Prof. Manfred von Ardenne
    - Intravenous injection of vitamin C and/or aloe vera
    - Find a practitioner who can help you to get off of as many medications as possible

14. Do not take cholesterol lowering drugs since they can kill you! People die of not enough cholesterol not from too much. This fact has been proven by medical doctor and professor, Walter Hartenbach. I will get to this later. (See the cholesterol hoax.)

15. Avoid all vaccinations. No vaccine has even been proven safe and effective. Plus, the toxins in the vaccine can cause autism, Parkinson's, Alzheimer's, cancer and even death.

16. Don't listen to the manipulation from the media, the pharmaceutical advertisements, or anyone around you who certainly means well but stands in your way of good health!

17. Throw out every energy drainer in your life—this includes negative people.

18. Stop all self-pity and don't let anybody pity you. This negative energy can kill you.

19. Make clear goals, both short term and long term. These should be inspiring goals that make you want to live and be healthy.

20. Create your own motivation as to why you want to live a long and fulfilled life.

21. Visualize yourself in perfect health and in a life that makes you happy. Imagine this in every detail as if it's happening right now. Experience, in your mind, how you are feeling and acting in your

happy and healthy life. Experience the things you are going to do in your future, things that inspire and excite you. As long as you cannot imagine yourself being healthy you don't have a big change of getting there. So train your imagination until you can visualize your future life in as much detail as possible. How do things feel? What sounds do you hear? What do you see around you? How do you look?

22. If you believe in God then spend some time each day in prayer. If you aren't sure of what to say, try this: *"Dear God, I thank you for my health and happiness, and for the healing that is taking place in my body right now. I am so grateful to know that You give me all of the answers and solutions I need so that I can achieve all of my goals for health, happiness and success."* Pray as if you are absolutely sure it is happening right now and will happen in the future without any doubts.

23. From now on use your common sense and your instincts when making any decisions. If it does not feel right, it is probably not right for you! I believe that our instincts are the voice of God within us. God speaks to us though our intuition and natural instincts. I believe that all illnesses are caused by our vibrations getting out of a healthy frequency because of our energy level being too low.

24. Recognize that you are the only one that has to live with the consequences of your actions, not your doctor who wants to put you through the torture of chemo and radiation, and not your relatives who have been brainwashed into believing that "poison, cut and burn" are the only chance you have of surviving.

   You have to answer to no one except yourself. This is why I cannot and will not make decisions for you. I can only educate you and give you my personal opinion based on my life experiences and observations, but you have to decide for yourself.

   At this point, if you still believe the medical route is the best option for you because you don't believe me or you don't want to take the responsibility for your own life and health and healing, then that is your choice.

25. After you read this entire book, take a few days off to think about it and to make up your mind. Take as much time as you need to feel sure about your decisions. Nothing is worse than doing something and not really believing in it, then having regrets later. I respect your decision either way, but please don't write to me later for help if you went the medical way, because by then it is probably too late.

26. Do not try both the natural and the medical route at the same time. In my experience every patient that did this died. Decide what you want to do and stick with it.

27. Do research and educate yourself.

28. If you don't have the money for all the supplements I mentioned, go on a 21 day fresh juice diet and organic raw food diet. After that, do the IBMS™ techniques and use all of the information in this book and pick at least one or two of the cancer fighters I've written about in these pages.

    Since I believe that all cancer is caused by mental and emotional stress, you should now be able to define and eliminate the root cause of your individual health break down and soon return to your normal state of health.

29. Recognize and accept that you now have: The Only Answer to Cancer! Your personal, individual answer! There is no healing power outside the body, only your own personal healing power given to you by Nature or God.

30. Never ever eat microwaved foods and protect yourself from EMC (Electro Magnetic Chaos) that is emitted from cell phones and computers. For extra protection, go to www.ewater.com for EMF

protection and cell phone boosters. Don't live underneath electrical lines since they cause cancer.

31. Do not get root canals with amalgam fillings since this is the main cause of breast and prostate cancer. Get all "silver" fillings in your teeth replaced with gold.

32. Underwire bras can restrict the lymph flow and cause breast cancer.

33. Do not watch TV, especially the news. Instead, become a member of Netflix or Blockbuster online and enjoy all types of movies, but skip TV, news radio and newspapers. That mindless propaganda will simply manipulate you and make you weak-minded.

Are You Worth It? Yes!

If you do all of the suggested things in this book, it is going to cost alot of money, especially when you look at it the very first time, but now let me ask you, are you not worth it? Of course you are! Good health is priceless. Who would be spending your money if you die from cancer?

Consider this an investment into your health and happiness. If you've worked hard all your life and have saved some money, now is the time to spend it on your future so that you can see your children and grandchildren grow up. Don't you want to live to do all the things you always wanted to do in your life? Don't you want to be with your loved ones as long as possible?

As I said, it is your life and your decision, but if you don't invest in your health and your life, then what is your money good for? Even if I didn't have much money, I would rather get into debt and get healthy, then pay it back later rather than die because of greed!

There Is No Such Thing As Cancer!

There is no disease called cancer, they just named normal natural occurrences in the body as such. And, if they would just leave it alone, most of the time it would simply disappear on its own the second the energy and nutrition, detoxification and hydration level is normal again. If you get rid of the root cause then you have no cancer symptoms!

Natural Proven Protocols From Around the World

Here are some of the natural proven cancer symptoms eliminators. Please note this is just a report for your personal research. If you use the listed proven, natural cancer treatments, you do it at your own risk. Also, you should ask an expert before and while you are following any of the following protocols.

1. The Eggplant cure from Australia
    This cure originated from the cattle herders of Australia. Dr. Bill Cham developed the latest cure for skin cancer—the Eggplant cure or BEC – 5. It is used successfully with basal cell carcinoma and squamous cell carcinoma without harming the skin in any way. I personally used to put my skin cancer patients into the sun and the sun cured in all my cases the skin cancer. Remember it's not the sun that causes skin cancer it's the sunscreen and/or environmental poisons and nutritional deficiencies. Dr. Cham's product is available at www.Cureaderm.net

2. The healing fruit from the Amazon
    Graviola or also called Guanabana, Annona or Brazilian Cherimoya is sold in local markets as fruit but used in many countries to successfully treat everything from diarrhea and dysentery to asthma and increasing the flow of mother's milk. It also has the proven ability to kill slow growing cancer cells. There are over 40 naturally occurring acetogenins in Graviola which have the strong ability to prevent abnormal cellular division which is the cause of cancer symptoms. Graviola has shown huge success with breast and colon cancer patients. Available from www.Rain-Tree.com Even Grapefruit juice has been proven to have a positive impact on cancer patients.

3. The tree that can make you happy
    The Chinese Happy Tree is used in China and Tibet for relieving depression and as a cure for everything from the cold and psoriasis, to liver, gallbladder, spleen and stomach diseases. It has been successfully used for ovarian and small cell lung cancers. It has also shown great results with metastatic colorectal cancer.

4. Cancer defying diet from Dr. Budwig
    The German doctor Johanna Budwig introduced to the world a nutritional package that successfully helped cancer patients fill in deficiencies and recharge nearly-dead metabolisms. The simple formula is based on omega 3 fatty acids and sulfur-rich proteins. Dr. Budwick's formula cured countless so-called hopeless cancer patients! The diet is based on flax oil and cottage cheese. Dr. Budwick found that a few simple foods can help fix the stagnated growth process in our cells. She found that when you combine flaxseed oil, with its powerful healing nature of essential electron–rich unsaturated fats, plus cottage cheese which is rich in sulfur protein, it produces a chemical reaction that makes the oil water soluble and easily absorbed into the cell membranes. Flaxseed oil has been proven to have a huge positive effect for patients with prostate, breast and skin cancer. Dr. Budwick uses 2 tablespoons of cottage cheese mixed with one tablespoon of flaxseed oil. The daily dosage is 6 to 8 tablespoons of flaxseed oil. People with pancreatic cancer have to work their way to this amount very carefully and slowly. Flaxseed oil can also help with arthritis, heart infarction and most cancers.

5. Acid-squeclhing combo from Dr. Hans Nieper
    My colleague Dr. Hans Nieper in Germany used an acid–squelching combo to enable the blood to repel cancer. Dr. Nieper cured countless cancer patients that I personally knew with cesium and DMSO treatments. Nature's most alkaline metal is cesium and when it is combined with DMSO it directly targets cancer cells, stopping the metastasis of the cancer, shrinking the tumor within weeks and

stopping the pain of cancer within 24 to 48 hours.

Dr. Nieper's protocol is: cesium chloride 1 – 6 grams a day. The usual dosage is 3 grams a day and always with food.

Breakfast: Cesium chloride (1 gram), vitamin C (1000 Milligrams), zinc (25 – 30 milligrams) one potassium capsule as prescribed by physician.

Lunch: Vitamin C (1000 milligrams)

Dinner: Cesium Chloride (1 gram), vitamin C (1000 Milligrams)

Before bed, after eating 2 slices of bread: Cesium chloride (1 gram) and vitamin C (1000 milligrams)

For purchase see:

www.rainbowminerals.net/cesiumPH.htm and

www.thewolfclinic.com/cesium.html

6. The detoxification cancer symptom cure named after Max Gerson: As the father of medicine Hippocrates stated so rightfully: Let food be your medicine, a German doctor Max Gerson did exactly that and invented a cancer detox diet today that still cures countless numbers of patients. His revolutionary diet is based on the philosophy that quickly revealed itself to be a potent nutritional and metabolic therapy and a cure for cancer!

For over 60 years doctor Gerson's diet has been based on organic fruits, vegetables and juices and helps detoxify the body quickly and effectively. It's helped countless cancer patients to completely recover from their cancer symptoms.

I believe that if you use Paul Nison's information you will also have great detoxification results. www.PaulNison.com You can also get more information about the Gerson diet from the Gerson Institute in Mexico 1-888-4GERSON. From inside the US call 619-685-5353

7. Mistletoe wiping out cancer symptoms

    The mistletoe has been used in Germany for hundreds of years to cure headaches, lung disease, internal bleeding, nervous conditions and cancerous tumors. It has the ability to help repair the DNA damage caused by cancer and to prevent the cancer from spreading. It has been successfully used to treat colorectal, stomach, breast and lung cancer. This treatment has to be injected and must be done by a physician because mistletoe can be toxic. It is marketed in Europe as: Iscador, Eurixor, Helixor, Isorel and more. For more information call: 800-241-1030 extension 5550 or go to www.weleda.com

8. Curcumin kills cancer cells

    Indian curries are a cancer blaster. The spice turmeric, whose main active component is called curcumin, is a well documented cancer fighter. It is a part of the ginger family and it's made by grinding the root of the large leafed Asian plant known as curcuma longa. Curcumin has been proven to inhibit a cancer provoking bacteria H.pylori associated with gastric and colon cancer. It can protect the DNA from damage and has been shown to be extremely effective with breast cancer, and it can protect you from radiation damage if eaten before x-rays. For more information call 800-877-2447 or go to www.Iherb.com

9. Ayurveda—herbal cancer fighting trio

    Triphala is a healing power source for reducing cholesterol, improving circulation, reducing high blood pressure, and improving liver function. It has anti-inflammatory and anti-viral properties and has been shown effective with pancreatic cancer. Triphala is the most popular Ayurvedic herbal formulas and it is easy for you to find information about this everywhere. It is taken as a tonic by stirring 2 or 3 grams of the powder into warm water and drinking it each evening. It is also available in capsules and is taken usually two tablets one or three times daily.

10. Cancer is a fungus

Dr. Tullio Simoncini from Rome, Italy has been curing cancer for over a decade with a simple solution of sodium bicarbonate (baking soda) and organic maple syrup. It is common knowledge in the medical profession that sodium bicarbonate can kill all sorts of fungi and microorganisms.

Dr. Simoncini has proven cancer is usually a Candida yeast infection (or always coexists with it).

Because the Candida acts as glue that keeps the cancer cells together, if you cure yourself from that fungus the cancer mass falls apart. The fungus produces an acid that is acid based and holds the cancer cells together. That is why it is so important to have an alkaline ph of 7.36 body environment.

Candida plays a vital role in the cancer's ability to survive, by making toxins that impair a cell's ability to self-destruct while allowing mutated cells to replicate into full-blown cancer. When Candida becomes intertwined with tumors, it stays alive along with the cancer.

This is why I had all of my patients do the
www.MyBePure.com
cleanse, the CandidaEX from
www.AwesomeSupplements.com
and take the silver from
www.HelpingAmericaNow.com .

I had such huge successes with prevention and cures of all kinds of cancer symptoms with just that trio of products, that they are a must for all my patients when it comes to cancer treatment and prevention.

Dr. Simoncini has had great success with his treatments in brain, bladder, breast, spleen, liver, lung, prostate, stomach, pancreatic and other cancers. Dr. Simoncini's protocol involves: 500cc of a 5% bicarbonate solution given intravenously over one hour six days a week or injected in localized, accessible tumors.

Today he has modified his protocol by alternating the bicarbonate injections with vitamin C intravenous injections. He also uses a mixture of sodium bicarbonate with organic maple syrup taken orally. Please read his book: *Cancer is a Fungus* and see www.CamelotCancerCare.com.

11. The macrobiotic diet for the fight against cancer
Macrobiotic literally means "long life" in Ancient Greek. The philosophy of the Macrobiotic diet is based on the idea of achieving balance for health and longevity. As I talk about all the time, health is a condition of balance. The Macrobiotic diet has been proven to cure cancer symptoms. It is based on dietary principles of simplicity, and avoidance of toxins that come from eating dairy products, meats and oily foods.

The basics are:
50% - 60% organically grown whole grains
20% - 25% locally grown and organically grown fruits and vegetables
5% -10% soups made with vegetables, seaweed, grains, and beans.

•   Other elements occasionally include some fresh white meat fish, nuts, seeds, pickles, Asian condiments, and non-stimulation teas.

•   Foods on the diet include vegetables such as potatoes, tomatoes, eggplant, peppers, asparagus, spinach, beets, zucchini, and avocado. It also advises against eating fruits that are not grown locally, such as bananas, pineapples, and other tropical fruits. The use of dairy products and eggs, coffee, sugar, stimulant and aromatic herbs, red meat, poultry and processed foods are to be avoided.

•   Clinical studies have shown that a low fat diet based on a foundation of whole grains, legumes, vegetables and fruit is the healthiest for cancer prevention and preventing the recurrence of cancer.

•   It has been very effective with pancreatic, lung, breast and colon cancer. This diet is low in protein, B12, iron, magnesium and calcium. I suggest supplementation.

12. The cancer fighting vitamin

For over 150 years the vitamin B17 (laetrile) had cured cancer symptoms! It is prevalent in bitter almond and fruit pits, mainly in the seed of Apricot. Laetrile is also known as amygdalin, originating from the seeds of plants in the prunus rosacea family and has been proven to cure cancer symptoms for centuries. It kills cancer cells without doing any harm to the healthy cells in the body.

Many doctors have used this with a near 100% cure rate. Please go to www.OasisOfHope.com and read *The Ultimate Guide to B17 Metabolic Therapy*. It should be taken with zinc, magnesium, vitamin A, E, B6, B12, folic acid and pancreatic enzymes. I personally get all my supplements from www.AwesomeSupplements.com

13. The cancer cure that may be gone soon

Antrodia camphorata is a cancer fighting Taiwanese mountain mushroom that has shown stunning results when it comes to cancer, as well as inflammation and toxicity. It has also proven effective in reversing and even destroying cancer cells. An added benefit is that it offers significant liver protection and can prevent or treat liver cirrhosis. It is extremely effective against liver cancer, bladder cancer, breast cancer, leukemia and lung cancer. It is often seen on the market under the name of Vitalsil.

14. Killing cancer with a poisonous plant

Oleander has cured advanced and inoperable cancer since the 8th century. It is also used to cure hangovers if combined with licorice. It has had stunning results with pancreatic cancer.

Oleander is available in capsules that are safe for human consumption. It is generally toxic, but in the right formulation it is deadly against cancer cells yet absolutely harmless to healthy body cells. You can also make your own oleander soup! Begin with ¼ to ½ of a teaspoon two or three times a day after meals. Work the dosage slowly up to 1 tablespoon three times a day after meals. For the full

recipe to create oleander soup visit my website at:
www.InstinctBasedMedicine.com.
Although you can make this soup, it is probably safer to research
where you can buy the capsules.

15. The injectable cancer cure

The Ancient Egyptians used aloe vera for cuts, burns and skin ir-
ritations. In 1930 it was used to treat skin irritation from radiation.
It also helps with constipation, psoriasis, frostbite, ulcerative colitis,
and diabetes. Injectable aloe is successfully being used to cure cancer
symptoms. The injectable form is called Albarin. It even helps to
limit the damaging effects of chemo or radiation therapy and helps
the body to heal and recover faster after surgery. The tumor shrinking potency has been clinically proven for a long time.
www.altcancer.com or call 877-737-6267

16. Cansema—and other secret cures

Cansema has been curing cancer since the 16th century, starting
with Paracelsus. It is made from "sal ammoniac" (ammonium chloride) along with fuligo (wood soot) and orpiment (arsenic sulfide)
to treat skin cancer and non-healing wounds.

By the way, a paste made from bloodroot, zinc, chloride, flour
and water was found in the 1900's to cure malignant growths and
generally destroyed the tumor within two to four weeks when applied directly to the skin cancer.

One native American cure for skin cancer is zinc chloride, bloodroot, bittersweet, ginger root, galangal and capsicum. This mixture
has been proven to destroy cancer cells without harming the healthy
cells. www.HerbHealers.com or 305-851-2308

17. The Canadian tea that has cured cancer for over 100 years.

A Native American concoction that has been used for many decades
by a nurse in Canada to cure cancers of all kind is called Essiac tea.

The success she has was so stunning that the governments did all they could to destroy the nurse, Caisse, and her formula.

The original formula included burdock root, slippery elm inner bark, sheep sorrel, Indian rhubarb root, watercress, blessed thistle, red clover and kelp. Over time it was later reduced to four mountain herbs: burdock root, sheep sorrel, slippery elm and Indian rhubarb. She named the tea Essiac, which is Caisse spelled backwards.

It has been so successful that I nearly always used it for my patients when it came to treatment and prevention.

www.AwesomeSupplements.com

This site has the Essiac Capsules that I found to be most effective.

18. Vitamin C—the super cancer killer

I personally nearly always used vitamin C in doses of 100 g per day and aloe injections intravenously in my clinics and Modern Therapy Centers™. I believe there is nothing more effective, safer and faster. Nobel Prize winner Linus Pauling called it Nature's Chemotherapy.

Vitamin C is the most important element in cancer cures since stress uses up huge amounts of this vitamin. Besides using my IBMS™ stress reduction CDs, you need huge amounts of vitamin C to combat the effects that stress has on the body.

19. Citrus Peels—the great cancer protection

Peels of citrus fruits like lemons, oranges, and grapefruit contain a compound called d-limonene which has been clinically proven to have a huge impact on a variety of cancer symptoms. It's especially useful in combating breast, skin, liver, lung, pancreatic and stomach cancer. The way it works is it causes apoptosis or, cell suicide of cancer cells. It is believed that it inhibits the ability of cancer cells to communicate with each other. www.lef.org or www.iherb.com

21. Oxygen—the force of life

Personally, I have used oxygen therapy in my centers. Manfred von Ardenne was the originator of this. This leads to an instant boost of energy and floods the blood with oxygen. The therapy is very simple. One quart of blood will be taken from the patient and intravenously put back after it was enriched with ionized oxygen. The energy boosting effects are instant and the healing effects kick right in. I have never seen any negative side effects with this therapy.

To recap what I've just said to you, as well as listing a few others, here is what I have witnessed as the best cancer cures:

- Hydrogen peroxide (35% food grade). I used 8 drops daily in 4 ounces of aloe juice
- Vitamin C injections
- Vitamin E - 400 IU for every 30 pounds of body weight
- Co-Q10
- Omega 3
- Thyroid support products (natural)
- L-cysteine
- N-acetylsteine
- Glutathione
- Burdock Root
- Essiac and Flor-Essence
- Oxygen treatments
- Flax seed oil
- Grapefruit seed extract
- All kind of organic fresh juices and fruits and vegetables

Of course, this is not all since we now know of over 300 natural cancer symptom cures. There simply isn't enough room in this book to talk about each and every one of them. I wanted to give you brief descriptions of the ones I feel are the best and that I have personally witnessed as beneficial.

For more information see my website
www.InstinctBasedMedicine.com

And remember, cancer is always stress related! If you get rid of the cancer symptoms without getting to the root cause of why you attracted cancer in the first place, it *will* come back!

A Note about Nurses

At this time I want to point out that when I show my utter disgust in regards to the medical and pharmaceutical industry that I don't include in this our wonderful nurses. They do all the work anyway and often know more about health and healing than doctors do. I also don't include in my disdain our experts in emergency and restorative medicine. These people are a godsend and we would not want to be without them.

What angers me are the MDs who hand out their dangerous toxins provided by the pharmaceutical industry.

When it comes to cancer; run as far away from the hospital as you can and get detoxified. Rebuild your own health and support your immune system as best as you can all through the power of God and Nature.

Another exception: Of course our doctors in the reconstructive and emergency field are the most competent and valuable MDs in the world. And that is the only field where the Medical profession has its true value! I admire their talent and their work.

Case Study of Healing with IBMS™
Healing of Bone Cancer

Gayle was a courageous woman who came to me with cancer that had spread into her spine, pelvis, and hips. She was referred from a renowned cancer clinic, as her doctor saw no possibility of helping her.

Gayle was energetic and committed to fighting for her health. She met all the prerequisites for my IBMS™ therapy. Gayle loved her life and career, had clear goals, and a healthy relationship with her children and husband. Initially, it was difficult to find a cause for what ignited this horrible cancer. The only thing I noticed was that Gayle became nervous when we discussed her previous relationships.

Gayle was so incredibly strong that it took four sessions to reach a breakthrough. She finally developed enough trust and rapport to tell me that she had been married previously. She was married to a gentleman from Turkey, who had convinced her to relocate there with vague promises and lies. Her life in Turkey was a living hell. Her mother-in-law abused and tormented her, and her husband treated her like an animal. This ordeal destroyed Gayle's personality. She started to isolate herself and withdraw. At times, Gayle was even suicidal. Her mother-in-law also tried to murder her. On a visit to Germany, Gayle visited a specialist who was supposed to examine and treat her because her condition had become life-threatening. During this visit, she successfully escaped from her husband and began a completely new life. Her health seemed to improve, but she repressed her past experiences and was filled with hatred toward her ex-mother-in-law and her former husband. She could not forget how she was abused, degraded and tortured.

Using the IBMS™ technique, I helped Gayle erase the past. She was stricken with cancer due to feelings of hatred, despair and helplessness. After ten appointments, Gayle could finally forgive her ex-husband and her former mother-in-law. She learned to accept them as they were and finally succeeded in letting go of these two people. Gayle also let go of her nervous responses whenever the past was mentioned. She also developed a new future perspective, as well as a new way of thinking that facilitated healing and recovery. Within four months, Gayle fully recovered. Today she is working full-time and is active, happy, and content with life.

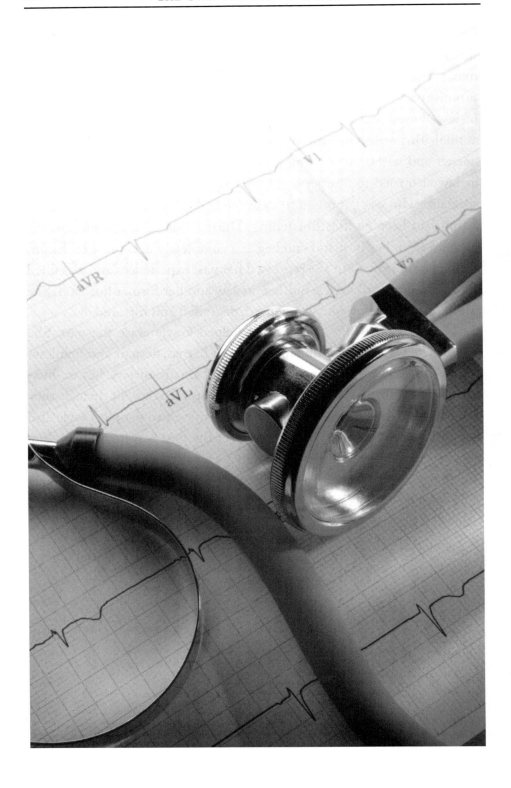

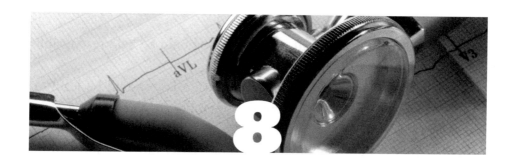

HOW I CURED MY PATIENTS IN EUROPE FROM ALL KINDS OF HEALTH CHALLENGES

From my mega best seller *The Great Book of Health*™, here are some summaries I want to share with you. You will find more information on my website www.InstinctBasedMedicine.com and on the CDs that were created to help you to apply all the knowledge in my books *Instinct Based Medicine* and *The Only Answer to Cancer* faster and much more effectively if you need or want to speed the IBMS™ process.

What is my goal with this book and all my work?
I will do everything in my power to achieve an amendment to the constitution for health freedom and patient rights and the full implementation of the constitution in general!

Historically, whenever the government interfered with mandatory health treatment—like leeching and mercury injections—it usually killed or at least potentially harmed the patient. Since the government is obviously practicing medicine without a license, every time they interfere with our health and treatment options, they should be held responsible their actions!

All humans should be created equal, so no law should be legal or applicable that makes any government member or persons or groups immune to criminal or civil prosecution. The only reason the government would do that is that they obviously know that criminal action will be committed and harm to the public will be done. Therefore, such laws should be voided and not acknowledged by any judge or jury.

The FTC, FDA and ACS are, in my opinion, only there to protect the interests of the pharmaceutical and medical industry. Therefore, it's a violation of their oath of office or given agenda and I believe it must be fraud, treason or some kind of prosecutable action. Any law that only benefits a few politicians or special interest groups like bankers, politicians and big money makers (pharma, oil, medicine, etc.) should automatically be null and void.

Since we are all equals shouldn't it be illegal to exclude anybody from the law or set them above it? Shouldn't the same laws pertain to everyone with no exceptions? Basically, as I understand the constitution with the right of freedom and liberty, we automatically have the freedom of choice for our own health and life!

If someone pushes mandatory vaccinations on us with proven toxins and harmful poisons and microbes, or forces mandatory chemotherapy, radiation or surgery that hurts and kills, doesn't it seem logical that the person or group or government or parts of it would be in violation of our constitutional rights?

Since all the facts about toxins and microbes in vaccines are well known and scientifically documented, and the effects of poisonous chemotherapy and cancer-causing and healthy tissue burning radiation are very well known, as well as the danger of surgery and related drugs, is it not an obvious conspiracy?

If what Dr. Tutto Simoncini says is true, the medical profession has a cancer cure rate of only 2% to 3% and yet cancer can be cured by over 300 natural treatments. The crimes against humanity are committed by the companies and politicians that are involved in the production and application of dangerous treatments and the political involvement of creating mandatory laws to apply these dangerous and killing treatments. Isn't this unconstitutional, maybe even treason, but at least a major crime? I think so!

Cholesterol is Good For You!

The money making and controlling scheme of the pharma and medical professions, in conspiracy with parts of government, are causing unnecessary illnesses and cancer and death by the minute! Cholesterol lowering medications will harm you and can make you die much earlier than you have to. It destroys the liver and/or kidney function. What's most scandalous of all is that there is no such thing as too high cholesterol! You die of not enough cholesterol.

Nearly 87% of all body cells are made of cholesterol. Every cell replacement therefore needs a huge amount of cholesterol! The production of hormones, your brain, and all of your body functions need cholesterol. The normal and average extremely healthy cholesterol level is 250 and above everything below 250 will create a problem for your body to function at an optimum level and to repair itself.

The conspiracy of the guys that make the big bucks on your suffering and the illnesses and symptoms they create by lowering your cholesterol is huge. They simply made up an unrealistic and unhealthy level of cholesterol and told you everything below 250 then above 200 and so on to make every person in America, or in the world for that matter, a patient! That is a horrific lie!

Cholesterol is good and there is no such thing as good cholesterol or bad cholesterol. LDL and HDL are not even cholesterol, they are transport proteins. Plus, nobody in this world has had a fatal heart attack caused by cholesterol. Every fatal heart attack has been caused by a chemical reaction (acidosis) and not by cholesterol.

Cholesterol is a good guy! It saves your life every single day! If you are toxic and are acidic that acid burns holes into your blood vessels. To avoid bleeding to death internally the cholesterol in your body goes there to clog the holes and stop the bleeding. If you have arteries that are clogged with cholesterol then you know that you have a heavy form of acidosis and should instantly work on it. I do the alkalizing protocol from www.AwesomeSupplements.com twice a year.

Salt and High Blood Pressure—Not True!

They tell you salt gives you high blood pressure because they know that if you don't have enough salt—at least half a teaspoon of sea salt or Stardust from www.GreatWholeFood.com--in your system you get sick or develop deficiency symptoms. You'll be chronically dehydrated, which is basically the main cause of aging, illness and cause of death. The fact is that most table salt contains many elements that are not salt at all such as glass or sand which cuts your arteries and the cholesterol now goes there to stop the bleeding. Because of that process, if it is all over your arteries it will raise your blood pressure, but it's certainly not the salt! So please use sea salt or 100% pure unrefined salt.

Eggs are good for you!

Everybody should eat at least 2 hard boiled organic eggs at least 4 times a week for good and healthy cholesterol levels. If you are on any kind of statin drugs, please find a licensed health care practitioner that will help you to get off of them ASAP! Every burn unit in every hospital I know gives their burn victims up to 20 hard boiled eggs a day because they know it is the fastest and safest way to rebuild healthy cells. So, if your money-hungry or incompetent MD tells you your cholesterol is too high, laugh at him and find a new physician. You can also write to me if you are looking for qualified help. Write to InstinctBasedMedicine@gmail.com

The Diabetes Fraud

Many colleagues of mine, countless therapists and researchers found that diabetes 2 can usually be cured by Eleotin and a vegetarian or raw food diet, along with a lot of water and enzymes. The Asian diabetes society and other organizations have called Eleotin (which is an herbal assembly and not a drug) the final cure for diabetes. It takes usually 1 to 5 months to cure the person, but this does work and I have seen this happen for many years!

High Blood Pressure—Easy To Fix

In my experience, high blood pressure can usually be easily normalized with full spectrum vitamin E, C and D plus Co Q10 and a raw food diet until it's normal. Of course, IV Chelation therapy is a huge help and is the fastest and most effective treatment I know. You still need the supplements above to keep it right, if you want my opinion on that. I have also seen patients completely ridding themselves of nearly every health condition by simply eating food from www.GreatWholeFood.com

Arthritis Usually Gone In 5 Months

I have seen many cases where arthritis, even rheumatoid arthritis, is completely gone in 5 months with the application of CMO and for the pain DMSO and for the inflammation hydrosol silver. Don't worry, I guarantee you will not turn blue like the "Blue Man" the media paraded so much some time ago! He caused it himself. You can listen to my radio show: http://www.blogtalkradio.com/TheDrColdwellReport or http://thedrcoldwellreport.blogspot.com and go to the archives and listen to that show about silver.

Most of all, listen to the shows: Instinct Based Medicine, Stress the Silent Killer and The Only Answer to Cancer. Here you will usually get all the information you need related to cancer or terminally illness on these shows.

Depression and Anxiety Cured—My Nearly a 100% Success Rate

The feeling of helplessness, hopelessness, feeling overwhelmed and living in fear without clear goals, action plans and lack of motivation, self-love or self-confidence and low self-esteem is usually the cause of depression and anxiety.

In my experience it is not a chemical imbalance that causes

depression, it is the state of depression symptoms that are causing the chemical imbalance. When I worked with patients, I used to give these missing elements, emotions and clarity to my patients with the same techniques that I used on my Depression and Anxiety research CD kit. This set consists of the Basic 3 CD IBMS™ stress reduction kit and these extra sessions: Take charge of Your Life, Bring Out The Champion, Life Solutions and Trauma Erase. The IBMS™ sessions are exactly what I used to train my patients' brains for total happiness and control. For more information visit www.InstinctBasedMedicine.com or write to me at: InstinctBasedMedicine@gmail.com

Vaccinations are an Assault with a Deadly Weapon

Vaccinations are, in my strongest conviction, the main if not only cause of autism, Sudden Infant Death Syndrome, Parkinson's, Multiple sclerosis, Alzheimer's and more. I'm certainly convinced that it causes cancer and most autoimmune diseases. The ingredients in vaccines are the most toxic elements found on earth!

List of vaccine fillers and adjuvants

You must first understand that an adjuvant is an agent that may stimulate the immune system and increase the response to a vaccine. This list, officially administered by design, with every vaccine provided to the public, in addition to the squalene that appears to be in this upcoming swine flu vaccine, is of great concern to many parents and grandparents. The first concern was the announcement that they would start vaccinating children and pregnant women first and then "wait to see if there were too many adverse events" (including seizures, neurological problems, and death). By the way, in countries that did not vaccinate against Polio, Chicken Pox and so forth, these diseases disappeared much faster than in countries that did vaccinate. Better hygiene and nutrition was the reason that these diseases would have disappeared anyway.

In addition to the viral and bacterial RNA or DNA that is part of the vaccines, here are the fillers:

- Aluminum hydroxide—directly linked to causing Alzheimer's disease
- Aluminum phosphate—directly linked to causing Alzheimer's disease
- Ammonium sulfate—an inorganic chemical compound used as a fertilizer and "protein purifier"; known to cause kidney & liver damage, and gastrointestinal dysfunctions
- Amphotericin B—an "antifungal disinfectant" and anti-biotic, which damages the urinary tract, bowels, and heart functions
- Animal tissues (a causal element for all the various auto-immune diseases associated with vaccination): horse blood, rabbit brain, dog kidney, monkey kidney, chick embryo, chicken egg, duck egg, pig blood, Porcine (pig) pancreatic hydrolysate of casein (the pig protein/tissue is an additional objectionable issue for Jewish and Muslim people)
- Calf (bovine) serum & fetal bovine serum (cow blood is recognized as a significant transmitter of Mad Cow Disease)
- Betapropiolactone
- Formaldehyde—used as "a preservative & disinfectant," known to cause cancer, chronic bronchitis, eye irritation when exposed to the body's immune system
- Formalin
- Gelatin
- Glycerol
- Human diploid cells (originating from human aborted fetal tissue)
- Hydrolyzed gelatin
- Monosodium glutamate (MSG) - now known to cause cancer in humans, also linked to obesity
- Neomycin (anti-biotic)
- Neomycin sulfate (anti-biotic)
- Phenol red indicator—a highly toxic disinfectant dye, attributed to liver, kidney, heart & respiratory damage

- Phenoxyethanol (antifreeze)—proven to have neurotoxic side effects
- Potassium diphosphate
- Potassium monophosphate
- Polymyxin B
- Polysorbate 20
- Polysorbate 80—associated with infertility when injected
- Residual MRC5 proteins
- Sorbitol
- Sucrose
- Thimerosal (mercury)—a neurotoxin linked to psychological, neurological, & immunological problems—especially autism. Nervous system damage (such as subacute sclerosing panencephalitis (SSPE), brachial plexitis, post-vaccinal encephalitis, transverse myelitis and peripheral neuropathies), kidney disease, birth defects, dental problems, mood swings, mental changes, hallucinations, memory loss, and inability to concentrate can occur. Symptoms also include tremors, loss of dermal sensitivity, slurred speech, and—in rare cases—even death and paralysis. This additive alone was the catalyst for another recent Class Action Lawsuit organized by mothers of children born with autism & the many related behavioral disorders associated with it. Autism is now occurring at levels never seen before in history; depending on the state, its rate is now 1 in 67 to 1 in 150. The autism rates used to be 1 in 20,000. Mercury may also be associated with the significantly increased rates of senility and Alzheimer's, which is associated with five or more successive flu vaccinations. Although most mercury (thimerosal) has been removed from children's vaccines, it is still in all flu vaccines at toxic doses.
- Tri(n)butylphosphate,
- VERO cells, a continuous line of monkey kidney cells - linked to the SV-40 virus known to cause leukemia
- Washed sheep red blood cells
  *This data is available via: www.mercola.com

http://articles.mercola.com/sites/articles/archive/2001/03/07/vaccine-ingredients.aspx

These additives are given to our children without public knowledge or consent and now your children have to be vaccinated to attend school or kindergarten! See www.nvic.org for qualified information.

How I Cured Skin Cancer in My Patients

Historically, after I had them complete what now is called the Be Pure Cleansing system, I flushed their mutated skin parts with sodium bicarbonate (baking soda) and put them on 25,000 IUs of Vitamin D3, three times a day and three times a day put them in direct sunlight for 12 to 20 minutes, directly on the skin where the mutations occurred. Plus, my general cancer kit, of course. For more specific info write to:

instinctbasedmedicine@gmail.com

or see

www.instinctbasedmedicine.com

How We Cured Colon Cancer

In my MTC (Hospitals) in Germany my employees or colleagues used, after a simple colon cleanse and the usual cancer supplementation, Oxygen Multi-Step therapy after Prof Manfred von Ardenne. I would also blow ionized oxygen directly on the tumor and often saw the tumor, the same way as Prof von Ardenne published in his works, that the tumor shrank in front of our eyes.

After that we flushed the colon with a sodium bicarbonate solution and usually had extremely fast success. We also used to have our patients sit in an oxygen chamber, no matter what their health challenges were, and this was a huge success.

The Swine Flu Crime

What in the world is wrong with so many Americans? Where is John Wayne when you need him? It's a proven fact that the swine flu vaccine has been created artificially in a lab and set free on purpose. They patented the brand new virus 2 years ago! Where did they even get the vaccine from for the flu?

Just a few (already sick) people died of the swine flu (if this is even true—there is no way to prove this after they are dead for 3 days) yet thousands die worldwide of the seasonal flu every year! Is this really enough to raise the pandemic level to 6 and basically order mandatory vaccinations for all member countries of the WHO? More people will die from the swine flu vaccine or get seriously ill, even though they never would have died from the swine flu. There are more dangerous toxins in the live virus vaccine than you could ever accumulate in an entire lifetime and it will harm everybody that gets the shot and kill many!

My Conclusion:

There are two reasonable questions that must be asked: (1) Is the swine flu live virus vaccine safe and effective, and if so, (2) will vaccinating 95% of the general population provide more protection for the whole population? If both of these questions were answered in the affirmative, then we would have a reasonable justification for mandatory vaccinations.

However, the overwhelming scientific data suggests just the opposite. The live virus swine flu is neither adequately tested, proven safe or effective, is non-insurable, and because of the well-known phenomena of Secondary Transmission aspects of a live virus vaccine, it may actually increase the transmission of the virus.

This live virus vaccine has 2.3 times more genetic mutability, and added adjuvant toxicity than a natural virus because it includes squalene. Squalene has significant autoimmune inflammatory effects, and general autoimmune effects, which are a potential significant threat to the health of the individual.

This is the most likely cause of the 300,000 GIs with Gulf War Syndrome who are applying for complete disability. All the scientific studies on the effectiveness of the flu vaccine to date show minimal to zero effectiveness. In other words, the benefit to risk ratio is extremely poor from a scientific point of view.

In answering the second part of the question, all the vaccine studies to date show that vaccinating 95% or more of a population did not make a difference in stopping outbreaks of a particular disease the people were vaccinated for. In fact, based on the scientific evidence, mass mandatory vaccinations with a highly mutable live virus could actually activate a real and lethal pandemic rather than prevent it. Therefore, from a purely scientific perspective, there is no valid scientific reason for mandatory vaccinations. For this reason we believe that all people have a constitutional, religious, and medical right not to be vaccinated against their will.

A summary

The overwhelming scientific studies and research do not in any way support the action of mandatory scientific flu live virus vaccination; to do so might result in the desecration of most of God's creation of humanity and planet earth; the science and destruction strongly suggests that mandatory vaccination are both immoral and ethically illegal (ethics that are core in the Judaic-Christian system and this mandatory vaccination violates the basic 10 commandments in 5 ways: Thou shall not murder, steal, lie or bear false witness, engage in idol worship (money and power), envy or covet.

> Liberty is to the collective body, what health is to every individual body. Without health no pleasure can be tasted by man; without liberty, no happiness can be enjoyed by society.
> –Thomas Jefferson

> Never doubt that a small group of thoughtful committed citizens can change the world; indeed it is the only thing that ever has.
> –Margaret Mead

For more information go to my friend Dr. Rima Laibows's website www.healthfreedomusa.org

Illness is based on lack of energy and that is to 86% cause by stress.

To protect my loved ones I would get the CD set from: www.instinctbasedmedicinestore.com and silver from www.helpingamericanow.com and the vitamin D 3 from www.awesomesupplements.com
For more and constantly updated information on all these issues see www.instinctbasedmedicine.com

Their Fraudulent Excuses

"There is no scientific evidence that shows that X causes cancer or any other diseases or illnesses…"

FTC, FDA, ACS, Media and other crooks use this completely absurd and scientifically stupid sentence to ignore or prove their lies about any cancer or illness causing facts. Like there is no conclusive scientific evidence that Fluoride causes cancer or there is no scientific evidence that vaccines cause autism. Of course not! Because the crooks that sell this junk are not conducting a study that would prove their poisons kill people and no one else has the money to do these studies. So of course there is truly no scientific study that shows that you are criminals because you protect each other and make sure that if a study comes out proving the truth that your products are killing people, you defame the messenger or create some kind of false evidence that the study is not reliable.

It really irritates me when I hear someone in the media saying the American Cancer Society says there are no scientific studies done that connect vaccines or mercury or chlorine and fluoride with the development of cancer, therefore there is no scientific evidence linking X to cancer. Or the other way around there is no scientific evidence that Essiac Tea, B 17 or vitamin D3 or vitamin C IV injections cure cancer symptoms—and that is a blatant lie.

They claim that they have the right to say what is scientific and what isn't! Their science has nothing to do with true science. So from now on if anybody ever says there is no scientific evidence or study that shows that X does XYZ—you know that they don't have the answer or know what they are talking about or they're just trying to hide the truth.

Here is what I wrote to President Obama and it's published on the

Obama support website.

Resolving the Health Care Crisis within 4 years
By *Dr. Leonard Coldwell* - Jan 17th, 2009 at 4:38 am EST
Comments | Mail to a Friend Report Objectionable Content

The Medical Doctor/ Medical Profession is the number one cause of death in America due to the hospital's medical errors and side effects of Pharmaceutical Drugs. This is the main cause of illness and permanent health limitations as well as chronic disease. I am convinced that the only way to resolve the Health Care Crisis is to change the education for Medical Doctors and to start educating the public in prevention and self help / self healing. As the leading authority for cancer and stress related illness and health education I can guarantee that I can fix the Healthcare crisis as well as the health care costs within 4 years if given full support. Please look at the facts that every cancer can be curable within 4 to 12 weeks if the patient did not have any form of chemotherapy, radiation treatment or surgery. I have proven that fact over and over again. If you are interested in the proof just read my newest book: Instinct Based Medicine How to survive your illness and your doctor.www.instinctbasedmedi-cine.com

    Respectfully,
—Dr. Leonard Coldwell

Yes, I could fix the health care crisis and get nearly everybody healthy within 4 years if I would be given the legal, political and financial power to do so. And after that prevention and education would keep at least 90% of the population healthy anyway and the health care costs would nearly disappear—except for accidents.

    Cancer, diabetes, heart related problems, arthritis and so much more can be cured with all natural extremely cheap treatments that have been proven safe and effective in many cases even for thousands of years. My colleagues and fellow researchers, friends and health freedom fighters can prove that any time. Just give me the authority and possibility to apply my system legally and give me 100 patients with cancer, diabetes 2, high blood pressure, or arthritis and I fix the problem in at least 90% of all cases within 2 to 16 weeks.

The Dr. Coldwell Diet for Weight Loss

Over the years I've found some weight loss strategies that have worked very well for me, my friends and my patients. If you'd like to lose some weight and *do not already have cancer*, my weight loss plan can help you shed some pounds in a short amount of time. For those who have been diagnosed with cancer, please see my website www. InstinctBasedMedicine.com for more information. **Note: Please talk to your doctor before going on any diet or weight loss plan.

1. For 2 days eat anything and everything you'd like. You'll be cutting out carbohydrates while on this weight loss plan, so enjoy some of your favorites.

2. Start the Be Pure Cleansing system from www.MyBePure.com

3. Do not eat anything for breakfast or lunch, drink filtered water or fresh juices only, and for dinner each night eat proteins such as steak, fish, eggs, and chicken. Do not have any carbs like pasta, rice or potatoes. Eat all of the vegetables you'd like, along with plenty of fresh salad with dressings made of olive oil, lemon juice, herbs and spices, or any low carbohydrate dressing. Eat as much as you want at dinner time.

4. Add herbs, spices, and sea salt to your foods as you wish.

5. Drink a gallon of filtered water each day with half a teaspoon of sea salt in it.

6. Prepare in advance for those times when you know you'll be hungry. I have my worst hunger pangs around 3pm so what I do is get busy! I run errands, work outside, or anything I can do to keep my mind

off of eating since I know I'll be having dinner at 6pm and can eat all of the protein and fresh veggies that I want. If you get hungry, keep yourself busy and within half an hour to 45 minutes your urge to eat will usually fade.

7. Don't eat after 8pm, tell yourself you have stayed strong all day long and it is not worth ruining your weight loss efforts by eating now. If I get very hungry and can't wait until morning, I have some pumpkin seeds. Just don't eat any sugary foods or carbohydrates. Stick with protein and vegetables only. After 3 days your cravings for sugar, starches and junk foods should disappear.

8. While you are on this weight loss plan, you really should take Quint-Essence from www.AwesomeSupplements.com to ensure you don't have any deficiency, or try the SynBioFood from www.Trinisol.com

9. If you mess up one day, that's okay! However, the very next day get right back on track as if you never went off your diet.

10. Weigh yourself every morning before you eat or drink anything and write it down to keep track of your weight loss efforts.

11. If you need support and strength to stay motivated, get the IMBS™ stress reduction CD package plus the mega-powerful weight loss CD. For information see www.InstinctBasedMedicine.com

12. After you lose as much weight as you'd like, you can go back to eating other foods. However, be sure to only choose what you really like and not what simply became habit. Another benefit to this diet is that you'll get full faster since your stomach will shrink!

13. For maintenance, if you gain 2 pounds just go back on the weight loss plan for a day or two—only proteins and vegetables—and that should take care of it.

14. For continued weight loss you can follow the insulin diet. What you do is eat any sugars, breads, carbs and fruits at breakfast time then eat nothing for 5 hours. For lunch and dinner have only protein and vegetables, making sure that your meals are 5 hours apart. Don't eat after 8pm. Most people still find that they lose about a pound a day even if they eat a huge amount of calories a day. A medical professor in Germany invented the insulin diet and has had huge success with it.

15. Find what works for you. I combined various things until I found what worked best for weight loss and optimal health.

16. If you need some help in losing weight, you can add Finally Slim from www.AwesomeSupplements.com; that helped me a lot.

17. I've also found that a 24 hour fast once a week is good in helping to shed extra pounds. Simply avoid food for one day each week and drink at least a gallon of water. Just doing this cuts down on 52 meals a year. Imagine the money you can save on food, and how good you will feel since your clothes won't be so tight anymore.

18. Don't eat anything you do not absolutely love! However, do eat in moderation. Eat only as long as you are hungry or have a craving. Once you've been satisfied, put the rest of the chocolate (or other goodies) into a ziploc bag or other storage container and put it away for later. You don't want to deprive yourself, but you don't want to be a glutton.

19. When you're hungry between meals have a big glass of water since this usually makes you feel full for awhile.

20. Play a game with yourself. When you're hungry say: "I'll see if I can wait another 15 minutes or half hour before I eat." Just try it. Many times the urge to eat will fade since most of us have programmed ourselves to eat even when we aren't really hungry!

21. Buy yourself a reward once a week or so. You may want to make this something you enjoy eating but don't normally buy for yourself. Try to make it something that's relatively expensive and decadent so you can have just a bite or two and you'll feel satisfied.

22. If you feel hungry and can't wait until your next meal, eat something healthy. Everyone can find a few healthy things they enjoy eating! When you weigh yourself the next morning you'll feel motivated when you see the scale going down.

23. Once a week try a juice fast. Drink only juices for one day. Again, go on a raw food diet for awhile. More information can be found here: www.PaulNison.com

24. Mix it up! See what works for you and what doesn't. That's why it's so important to weigh yourself every morning. Keeping a journal can help track your progress as well.

25. This is not a scientific diet or concept; this is just something I've witnessed over time that has worked for me and many other people. So don't be too strict with yourself or too hard on yourself. Use your instincts and discover what works for you.

26. Play with it and have fun. "Gain a pound of Health, Happiness and Vitality™ with every pound you shed!"

I've just provided many suggestions that have worked for me, my friends, clients and family members. I'm not telling you that you *should* follow any health plan. You need to find your own answers to weight loss and health. If in doubt, before you start any diet, see a health care professional.

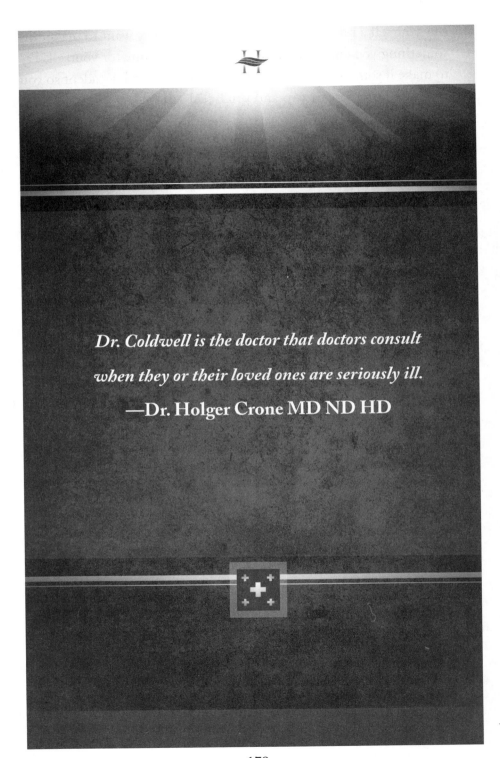

Dr. Coldwell is the doctor that doctors consult

when they or their loved ones are seriously ill.

—Dr. Holger Crone MD ND HD

PART 2

ANSWERS
FROM WORLD
EXPERTS

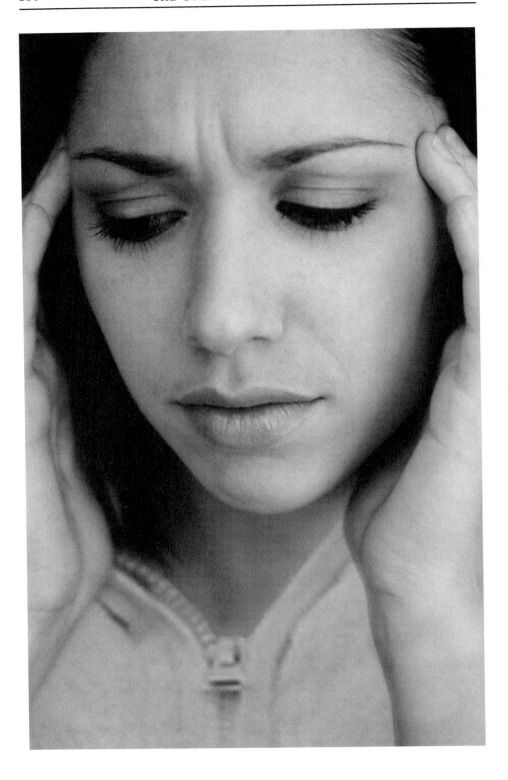

CANCER, THE TEACHER

RIMA E. LAIBOW, MD

In 1994 I woke one morning and instead of my usual good morning kiss to Bert, my beloved husband, I said, "You have terminal prostate cancer." He replied, quite naturally, "Well, good morning to you, too!"

Even though I know how important intuition, or non-linear information access, is, I realized how weird this must have sounded to Bert, because it certainly sounded weird to me. I also knew that not following up on information like this could be a fatal mistake. I told Bert that we would use conventional allopathic techniques to find out if I were really in touch with accurate information or just had an underlying resentment I was not aware of toward him!

My definitive words touched off a justifiable panic in him not only because of the deep terror that "cancer" can strike in the heart of so many people, but also because his father had, like so many elderly men, developed prostate cancer for which he was surgically castrated. Before I met my husband and his family, they had decided that the advice of the Army doctor caring for his father, a retired career Army officer, was necessarily correct because he was, after all, the doctor and in their world of hierarchical thinking, if a superior figure said something, it must be true.

Therefore, the family did not look for alternatives to this mutilating surgery. They did not use the Internet or the library for information on what else they could do. They saluted and said, "Yes, Sir!" to the offer of this barbaric surgery.

Surprisingly to the family and to his father, Bert's father began to vanish before their eyes. He shrank physically and shriveled mentally since the testosterone necessary to maintain both physical and psychological vigor vanished abruptly. Bert had described it to me as watching his beloved larger-than-life dad vaporize before his eyes, loosing his zest for living, his love of the outdoors, his vitality and his mental clarity. He no longer needed his testicles for reproduction, but he certainly needed them for vital living.

So my words opened the abyss in front of Bert's eyes with a quick slide into passionless oblivion on top of a life-threatening disease.

We rapidly sought out medical services to run blood tests for hormones and perform an ultrasound. Both showed strong evidence of my accuracy—which I hoped would be tossed into a cocked hat. We were advised that a needle biopsy was important to stage the cancer and assist us in making plans for treatment, or worse. We declined emphatically and, at least initially, politely since I was well aware of the potentially disastrous seeding of cancerous cells in the needle track once a malignant lesion is entered and withdrawn from by a needle during the course of the biopsy.

I had been in medical practice for 24 years at that point using only drug-free methods to treat and cure my patients. While never a believer in the official line about much of anything's, I was, as I still am, in evolution. Just a day or so before I had said to Bert that although I knew that cancer chemotherapy and radiation were ineffective, mutilating, primitive and brutal, I wondered whether I would have the courage to use other methods if I were personally faced with cancer.

Once that reality stared me in the face, the reality was very different.

I was totally confident that conventional burn, slash and poison treatment was wrong. I can only assume that the assurance I felt came from the same place as the diagnosis.

I proposed to Bert that we not use conventional treatment but instead "do something smart and use natural treatment." Given his personal history with the impact of conventional treatment, it is not hard to imagine the vigorous enthusiasm with which he agreed to do whatever I thought best.

Cancer indicates immune failure

My approach was simple for this, my first natural cancer treatment case: I realized that cancer was not an organ-based disease, but a specific indication of a generalized immune failure manifesting in a particular organ which was fundamentally toxic (or anti-nutritional) and nutritional in its origin and causation. Therefore, since Bert had no symptoms of the disease, I ignored it and concentrated not on the disease but on the underlying cause of the disease.

I created a protocol which consisted of every natural, non-toxic immune booster of which I was aware at that point in my development. I used large doses of organic, pure nutrients like curcumin, the active ingredient in turmeric, Co-Q-10, zinc, Vitamins A, B (all, with the exception of Vitamin B 1, Thiamin, which can act as a growth promoter), C, D, E. If I had had a source for Laetrile, sometimes called Vitamin B17, I would have included that as well. We included Poly MVA and the associated, vile tasting, but important Tibetan herbal formulation. Resveratrol, germanium sesquioxide, medicinal mushrooms (Maitake, Shitake, Reishi and others), biotin, mixed natural carotinoids, biotin, selenium, grape seed extract and other antioxidants, abundant probiotics, pre-biotics, adrenal support, whey protein isolate, saw palmetto, pygeum, high quality fish oil, a highly alkalinizing diet and plenty of betain hydrochloride, DGL plus a modest amount of copper were all part of the mix. So was a totally organic diet, rich in green drinks but without any added sugar or high sugar foods, plenty of pure, clean water and an abundance of love, laughter, meditation, visualization and joy.

Bert was taking two large handfuls of supplements, herbs and nutrients every day. After about 4 months of this regimen, he started grumbling and complaining about the amount of "stuff" he was taking. I must admit that I smiled sweetly and said, "That's OK, Darling! You don't have to take any of this anymore. We can treat you the way your dad was treated." He immediately stopped whining about the regimen and complied beautifully.

After 8 months, his markers were all back to normal and there was no sign of cancer. I reduced most of the input and after 4 more months, all markers of every system were not only normal, but optimal. Today, 15 years later, Bert is hale, hearty and vigorous. He is, of course, cancer, heart disease, arthritis, diabetes, and other disease free.

Bert was my first cancer patient and I was determined to throw everything I could at the cancer because my love's life was at stake. I realized that this would make it impossible for me to know with certainty what had been the responsible curative agent, if, indeed, there was one.

Once I found myself immersed in a life-or-death battle with cancer using only natural tools, I realized that while the kitchen sink filled up with everything I could think of was a good first step (and worked magnificently), I needed to get a lot smarter to confront cancer in a much more effective, efficient and cost-effective way.

Things I learned and practiced

I learned, and became certified in, chelation therapy to remove the heavy metals associated with cancer, referring to biological dentists to remove amalgams carefully since weakened immune systems dealing with the continuing onslaught of mercury, lead, cadmium, beryllium and other heavy metals are staggering under loads that make recovery difficult or impossible.

I learned about high dose vitamin C and mineral drips and saw the benefits with my patients of intensive cellular nutrition using 100 grams of Vitamin C plus high levels of associated nutrients including, of course, high levels of selenium, 3 to 5 times per week.

I learned that, at least for my cancer patients, a high percentage of raw organic food in the context of a totally vegan diet using healthy fats and oils in good supply was an essential component of recovery since the arachadonic acid (AA) found in animal products can act as a promoter for cancer cells. Mucus producing foods allow the cancer cells to "hide" in glycoprotein coats so they have no place in the diet, along with pro-inflammatory foods or high-sugar foods. No sugar, no white flour and no dairy, not even organic, unless the milk is organic and raw, are essential rules for cancer patients.

Detoxification is an obvious and vital pathway to recovering immune competence so I became an Environmental Physician by taking the outstanding training offered by the American Academy of Environmental Medicine, www.AAEM.com and the American College for the Advancement of Medicine, www.ACAM.org. I installed a far infrared sauna in our office with a shower and brought in a highly skilled lymphatic massage therapist to assist in detoxification as well as a "bounce chair" to move the lymph prior to sauna therapy, using nutrients to increase GI detoxification at the same time.

DMSO, that remarkable molecule which increases immune function and penetration of nutrients, in an IV solution following a nutrient IV proved useful to large numbers of patients although it can be hard to find a medical grade product and it is not safe to use any other type IV.

Nutritional products like whey protein isolate to deliver high oral levels of glutathione, the body's primary antioxidant, alpha lipoic acid, Halen, an organic fermented soy drink from China which "tricks" the cancer cells into ingesting substances which are toxic to them, but beneficial to normal cells (but which tastes and smells really, really awful) proved useful with some patients. The trick, of course, was to determine which regimen suited the nutritional, clinical, emotional and physical situation of each patient.

Case in point

Sometimes simple, intensive nutrition alone was life saving. For example, one Friday afternoon when the staff had worked particularly hard during the work and we had no late patients, I gave the staff the rest of the afternoon off and we were closing up the office. My nurse looked out the window and asked if we had an appointment with a patient in an ambulance. We looked blankly at one another for a moment and then rushed to check the appointment book since we all realized that we might have overlooked someone's appointment. There was, however, no one on the calendar.

By this time, the elevator doors opened and a very ill young woman with tubes in every possible location was wheeled though the office doors on a gurney, pushed by 3 ambulance attendants and flanked by her distraught mother, father and husband.

The story was a tragic one: this 44-year-old mother of 2 young children had been diagnosed with a highly aggressive stomach cancer which had led to metastatic disease in her abdomen and elsewhere. A procedure had been recommended after the chemotherapy and radiation had failed but the HMO wanted to pay for it only at the cheapest price possible. They spent weeks looking for a discount and finally sent her to Mary Hitchcock Memorial Hospital in New Hampshire from her home in Southern New Jersey, a 14 hour drive, strapped on her back in an ambulance.

When she arrived at the hospital, they examined her and said that she was too far advanced now and told her family to take the unconscious woman home. They asked if she could spend the night in the hospital since the trip was so hard on her but since her HMO would not authorize a night in the hospital and ordered the ambulance to make the round trip immediately.

They pulled into our office about 2.5 hours from home and asked if we could help their wife and daughter.

After taking a history I realized that she was being fed sugar water, the best food available for her cancer and the least effective for whole body, let alone immune, nutrition. I mixed up some very high potency IVs, explained to the family that they were to hang a bottle every 12 hours around the clock, gave them my phone number and told them to call me if anything changed. Otherwise, they were to come to see me first thing Monday morning.

None of us expected to see her again. On Monday morning, however, bright and early, there she was, in a wheel chair, to be sure, but smiling, bright eyed and beaming. Clearly, nutrition was an essential issue here so I began treating her with very high potency nutrients on a daily basis, using the established IV access to allow her to be treated at home, but under my care.

The next weekend was Memorial Day Weekend and she declared that she was ready for a party: she was pain free, her body had begun to eliminate waste again and she felt like dancing! And dance she did, while about 150 people celebrated her return to life.

Two days later, she attended the flute recital of her two daughters, free of pain and full of joy.

The story goes downhill from there. She had been producing 6 liters (1.5 gallons) of fluid generated by the cancer cells in her abdomen every single day. It was drawn off with a large syringe. As she got better, the amount decreased until, when she visited her cousin, who was also her doctor, he was amazed to find that he could only draw off 20 cc (0.02 liters). He examined it with his naked eye, not bothering with a microscope and decided that since the fluid was cloudy, it must be infected. He had, in fact, never seen the breakdown products of a tumor in the process or resolving and so had no frame of reference for a healthy patient producing cloudy ascites fluid.

Despite the fact that she was fever free, feeling wonderful and full of energy, he proceeded to treat her for the infection that he was convinced she must have and gave her vancomycin, a highly toxic antibiotic, absent any testing of her liver functions or attempt to culture the fluid to see if there were organisms in it.

Her liver, weakened and damaged by the chemotherapy she had survived, could not tolerate the toxic compound and she died following the initial treatment with the vancomycin. We cried at her funeral with her family.

Cancer is a complex disease with multiple causes and multiple approaches to reverse and repair its damage. All cancer treatment centers around the immune system, its nutrition and its integration into a healthy matrix. High doses of enzymes, for example, are essential in solid tumors while adult stem cell preparations allow repair cells to circulate without the risks, dangers and failures of stem cell transplants.

But there were other tools to help deal with the immune system failures and emotional issues—always critically important—for each patient. Frequency medicine, including diagnosis and treatment centering on the information found in the voice of each person became very important to us.

Voice Analysis

An example: a woman came to our office because of pervasive and unrelenting fatigue and malaise. I decided that a voice analysis was in order, along with laboratory tests. Our procedure was that the person doing the voice analysis had no clinical information about the patient so that their interpretation of the voiceprint would not be biased in any way. Bert took the woman's voiceprint and looked at those frequencies most out of balance. Checking the database, he asked the patient if any of the four chemical names associated with those out of balance frequencies meant anything to her. She immediately burst into tears, to the astonishment of Bert-the-technician. He came to get me and I interviewed the patient, from whom I had not yet taken a detailed history.

It turned out that she had been in her horse paddock when her neighbor sprayed his orchard with those 4 chemicals. Her dogs had died, and she and her horse had rapidly developed cancer. Following the chemotherapy, she had never been well. The spraying and cancer treatment took place 15 years before.

We used frequencies specifically designed to detoxify those chemical residues from her system using her tone box at home: she rapidly became robustly and radiantly well.

In patients with active cancer, our approach was similar, but carefully tailored to the individual toxicities of the patient. We often also used the frequency of chemotherapy agents to deliver the impact, but not the toxicity, of the agent. This treatment was delivered through headphones plugged into a tone-generating box which we can program to deliver specific medicinal tones to the patient for specific time periods each time the box is used.

NeuroBioFeedback

NeuroBioFeedback is a frequency treatment in which the brain's own frequencies of activation (as seen in the EEG waves) are measured and information about them is fed back to the patient through sound or light on a computer monitor when the brain improves its frequency function. No input is made directly to the brain; only reward information is presented when the brain does more of what you want it to do. In cancer, there are profound changes in brain function since the immune system is regulated "from above" and reversing those changes toward optimal states results in a major up-regulation of immune function and an equally major up-welling of the emotional issues buried in, and expressed through, the cancer. Concomitant psychotherapy and processing is absolutely essential for the detoxification of the emotional toxins which set the stage for, and continue, the cancer. In this, of course, cancer is not a unique disease since it is both intuitively obvious and scientifically increasingly clear that there is no meaningful distinction between the emotional body and the physical one. Both interact fluidly with one another and each impacts the other profoundly. Disorder in one is eventually reflected in disorder in the other so awakening the capacity to readdress trauma and emotional misinterpretation is essential to capture or recapture total health and radiant well being. Part of my intake interview with every patient with a chronic disease was to ask the question, "What will you loose when you are disease free?" The answers, after initial protestation that there was nothing to loose, were both revealing and orienting in where our further discussions needed to go to be maximally helpful. The second question I always asked was "What is the gift this disease has given to you?" Again, the dialogue was usually preceded by denial of any value or precious gift. With a little time and open listening, however, another level of reality opened and we could move forward with important emotional work.

Oxidative treatment

Other helpful frequency tools include a device which emits the frequency of ozone (O_3), but not ozone itself. Ozone is well known as an effective and powerful oxidative treatment for cancer but since it is so effective, but pumps no money into the coffers of Big Pharma, its use in many states is cause for loss of a doctor's license. Since there is no prohibition on providing patients with the active principle of ozone, its frequency, I felt comfortable doing so without fear of loss of my license. Indeed, using this device, I literally witness tumors the size of grapefruits shrink within an hour to a golf ball sized lesion. Further treatments totally eliminated the lesion and neither the patient's radiologist nor her other specialists were able to find any evidence of a tumor following about 2 months of treatment. Usually we combined this treatment with nutrition and detoxification for outstanding results.

Conclusion

At no time did I ever treat a patient's cancer. Every treatment was focused on either keeping the patient comfortable, if the underlying disease was causing pain or other physical problems or removing the underlying source of immune dysfunction, and correcting it. No state official ever tried to attack my license. No malpractice action every raised its head to threaten my practice. In fact, since my malpractice company informed me that they would not cover any aspect of my practice since I was not using drugs, I dropped my coverage, going "bare," and informed my patients of the fact that I had no malpractice coverage so suing me would not do any good if there were any dispute about treatment and I therefore encouraged them to bring any differences, discontents or problems directly to me so we could solve them together. They did and we did. They also signed clear, strong waivers stating that since I was not a Board Certified Oncologist, I was not treating their cancer, had not promised them a cure and was "only" offering immune support. That "only" meant that for large numbers of people, their cancer could not hold out in the face of renewed immune competence. We rejoiced together, but I did not take the credit. Their perseverance and dedication allowed them, like Bert, who took huge handfuls of pills and changed his diet drastically, to rebuild a depleted or damaged immune system, confront old devils and make a new start at life.

These brave and persistent people, usually arriving at my office in a state of terminal illness, have been among my greatest teachers and inspirations. I am grateful to all of them, starting with Bert, for offering me the gift of helping them heal.

In health and freedom,

Dr. Rima

Rima E. Laibow, MD

Medical Director

Natural Solutions Foundation

http://www.GlobalHealthFreedom.org

August 11, 2009

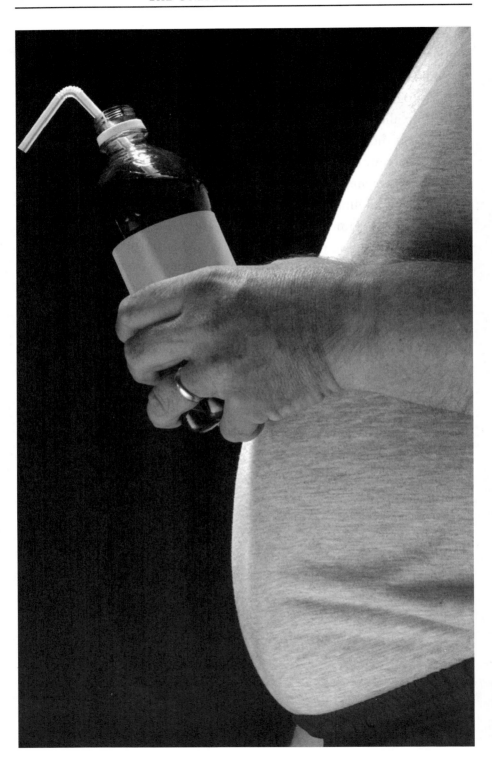

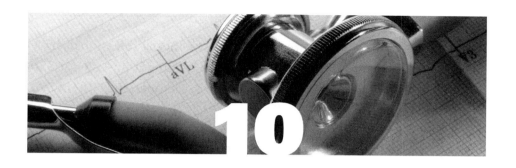

ARTIFICIAL SWEETENERS CAUSE CANCER

DR. BETTY MARTINI

It's 2 PM. Since midnight 850 Americans have forfeited their lives to the scourge of cancer that rages across our land. Before this day ends another 550 will perish, 1400 each day, 10,000 every week, half a million a Year!

Almost 50 years ago President Nixon declared war on cancer. So now it's right to ask what ground has been gained? What victory has been won? What have an Army of oncologists, a Mountain of machines and medicines and a river of money bought for us? Have they washed away the dread threat of malignancy that shadows America? The experts give the answer: The victory belongs to cancer! Year by year the numbers climb, there's more than ever before. Your odds of getting it are down to 1 in 3, they say.

Something else has grown, too. It's been said that there are as many people making a living off cancer as are dying of it. And a very good living it is for many doctors of death, and evidence is that their prime motivation is to maintain employment. These cancer Professionals have hijacked the health of our nation and they're holding it hostage for $80 Billion a Year. To the hostages, you and your loved ones, they offer but a bitter choice: Pick your way to die!

Butchery—The old favorite, we call it Surgery

Burning—Very modern and Hi-tech, Radiation Therapy

Poisoning—A specialty of the house, otherwise known as Chemotherapy

My Mother, Eve Geller, picked all of them and died after two years of horrible agony. It began with a small nodule in her right breast. She died a week after her final surgery, a hysterectomy. At the same time my best friend's mother diagnosed with breast cancer. The MDs said she would die in 6 months if they didn't operate. They operated. Susan Shuman refused surgery and survived 10 years!

In 1969 Hardin Jones PhD, a professor of medical Physics and Physiology at the University of California at Berkeley, declared: "For the typical type of cancer, people who refused treatment live an average of 12 years. Those who accepted surgery and other kinds of treatment lived an average of 3 years. I attribute this to the traumatic effects of surgery on the body's natural defense mechanism. The body has a natural kind of defense against every type of cancer."

In 1977, Dr. Jones reported that a woman with breast cancer who had no treatment lived up to four times longer than one who was treated by conventional methods. Dr. Alan Levin, of the University of California, San Francisco, confirmed this in 1987.

Most cancer patients died of chemotherapy. Chemotherapy does not eliminate breast, colon or lung cancers. This fact has been documented for decades. Women with breast cancer are likely to die faster with chemotherapy than without it.

In 1993, the October 4 Newsweek wrote: "Americans of any given age are as likely to die of cancer today as they were in 1971." That's when the war on cancer began. So 22 years, 10 million lives and a Trillion Dollars later, the cancer doctors, in a state of hypnosis, butcher, poison and burn us into early graves, inflicting heinous torture, death and destitution unequaled since Nazi death camps, and what have we learned? Only that their methods don't work! Today, in 2009, it's much worse with the continuation of approval of carcinogens like aspartame (NutraSweet/Equal/E951/Canderel, etc.).

The FDA revoked the petition for approval because it caused brain tumors and brain cancer, but Don Rumsfeld, CEO of Searle at the time called in "his markers" and got it approved anyway. In 1987, FDA toxicologist, Dr. Adrian Gross told Congress that aspartame violated the Delaney Amendment because of the brain tumors, and therefore how could they establish a safe dose. Delaney forbids putting anything in food you know will cause cancer. Dr. Gross' last words to Congress were, "If the FDA violates its own laws then who is left to protect the public?"

Today, half the population is using an addictive, excitoneurotoxic, genetically engineered, carcinogenic drug masquerading as an additive. Two Ramazzini Studies in Italy have proven again what the FDA knew three decades ago: that aspartame is a multipotential carcinogen.

The question is: Will A Cure For Cancer Ever Be Found?

And the answer is: Long Ago! But let me tell you a story.

It's a bright autumn day, the German time of Octoberfest, a season of harvest and holiday when the crop is gathered, the yield is tallied, and profits are counted.

Return with me now over 50 years to a Bavarian October in a little town not far from Munich. Munich, the ancient illustrious center of science, progress and education. Around you the mountain crags crowned with castles give assurance that you and your family are protected and safe.

However, your government has built nearby a city within a city, mysterious and private, fenced and walled, guarded with zeal by the Nazi SS, and to this desolate place go forlorn trains with sealed cars. You've learned the cars are crowded with People, helpless people. And when the morning mists cover the valley mingled with smoke from the camp furnaces, an evil scent, the aroma of death permeates your homeland. You try to ignore it, but you know that no one ever leaves that place, the cars are always empty; for you live in Dachau, destination of the damned, where torture, insanity and death rule as kings. Where medical experimentation is conducted, new toxins and antitoxins tried out, surgical techniques devised, and studies are made of the effects of artificially induced disease, all by experimenting on living human beings! And they all died, everyone died eventually. The bitter trains had one destination only: extinction. Destination extinction!

The problem of cancer has been solved, many times, but you and I are prisoners. We are in Dauchau. God's anger must rise up in his nostrils as he beholds entrenched financial empires filled with greed systematically denying lifesaving remedies so that millions die in horrible agony. It's genocide! We read at 1 John 3:17: "Whoever has this world's means for supporting life and beholds his brother having need and yet shuts the door of his tender com-passions upon him, in what way does the love of God remain in him?" Cancer is curable. It's time to burn the box cars and FREE THE PEOPLE.

The Eve Geller Memorial Cancer Formula:

My mother, Eve Geller, died a horrible death from cancer. I've never been able to get it out of my mind. Where did this formula come from that I've given out freely in my mother's name?

A friend of mine, Diane Murphy, was diagnosed with a rapidly spreading melanoma. After two biopsies the surgeon began to frighten Diane saying if she wasn't operated on quickly she would die. Diane met someone who had cured her melanoma naturally, and she gave Diane the name and address of Jettie, an aged woman who cured cancers ever since as a young woman she had married a Choctaw Indian.

The herbs cured Diane, but to be sure she decided to go to an internist. He refused to believe she ever had cancer and was totally against what he called "folk medicine." We asked the first doctor to please confirm with the internist that she had really had a large melanoma. Finally the internist called Diane and asked her to return to the surgeon who had assumed that she had died. When you have cancer they tell you you're going to die without them; when you cure it naturally they say you never had it in the first place.

Several years later, in fact 25 years to the day after Eve Geller died, I had a mammogram because of pain in my right breast. They found a nodule, as had initiated my mother's ordeal and death. It began to indent like in my mother's case. The surgeon told me "we'll take this out next week." My husband warned that if he penetrated the nodule, opened it up, it could metastasize and spread throughout my body. Also, I couldn't forget the horror that had been inflicted on my mother, so I declined, which infuriated the doctor. He hammered at me "this will never go away" and ranted until he brought me to tears, then flounced out of the room.

The nodule is gone now, these 18 years later, thanks to natural remedies. So I tried to find Jettie, the woman with the formulas, but she had passed away. Fortunately Diane Murphy remembered Jettie's best friend, Mary Henry. When we found Mary she said indeed she had the formulas, which had saved her life. Her story was like mine: her mother died of breast cancer and when Mary turned 30 she too was diagnosed with it.

Jettie had given her three formulas at that time and Mary cured herself, and then put the formulas in a safe where they remained for 30 years. I had asked Mary why she had not shared them, and she said she had offered many times but her friends wouldn't try it, chose chemotherapy and died. Mary said if I didn't charge large amounts for the formula she would fax it to me in the morning. I said that in Gen 1:29 Jehovah God gave us all green vegetation, and nobody should have to pay for the cure for cancer.

My breast had become very painful and indented, but after finally finding all the herbs and preparing them I started to use Jettie's formulas. Then one day the pain disappeared and my breast returned to normal. I wanted the world to have the formula but knew I could never market it because if there is one thing the FDA doesn't want cured is cancer. So I decided to name the formula for my mother and give it out to anyone who wanted it.

Shortly after I regained my health I met Eva who told me, tearfully, that she had been diagnosed with ovarian cancer, and who would raise her two young children? I gave her the preparations, and when she returned to her physician he said, "Eva, your cancer is dying." Finally when he could find no trace of cancer he requested that she have a hysterectomy. He said as a physician he didn't know if it was still in the tissues and after all she had suffered from endometriosis. I told her I couldn't make that decision for her, it was between her and her physician. So Eva checked into the hospital and the next day when I went to visit her she was packing. She said, "The doctor just left. He said to tell you that not only is the cancer gone but so is the endometriosis. He decided not to do the hysterectomy. This was about 15 years ago and Eva got to raise her children and is still going strong.

So began a journey of watching people with cancer return to normal healthy lives. Next it was Bob O'Neill, related to my husband. He had had prostate cancer for ten years and his physician said without surgery there was nothing left. Bob had been visiting and said he would die before having the surgery. Because physicians don't like so-called "folk medicine," Bob didn't tell him he was using the herbs. Months later his physician said, "Bob, I can't find the cancer." Cousin Bob has a great sense of humor and said, "Where do you suppose it went, Doc?"

The FDA's Control

It's important to know how far the FDA goes to prevent people from using natural remedies. One friend, Brenda, decided to use the formula for her breast cancer. One of the hardest ingredients to get is iodine, so she ordered it from Switzerland. It was confiscated in the mail by the FDA.

Once you could buy quinine sulfate at the drug store. Now it's only by prescription, but the FDA says it must be prescribed for malaria. Simply a capsule of this product is used in a Jettie's formula.

Next FDA put black snakeroot on the confiscation list. We bought several of the ingredients from an herbalist who grew herbs like his father before him. What the FDA did is just an abomination. One day when he was away the Government illegally sprayed his herbal gardens, acres, and killed everything. In small towns everybody knows everyone else. One of the Forestry team, before he died, told the farmer: "The FDA made us do it. They said herbs were unsafe."

Now let's get this straight: FDA blesses aspartame, a deadly addictive, excitoneurotoxic carcinogenic drug that not only triggers birth defects without a warning on the label and for which FDA has received more volunteered complaints than any other food additive in history. This chemical is not only a multipotential carcinogen, but breaks down to DKP, a brain tumor agent. It triggers multiple neurodegenerative diseases so in 1995 FDA listed 92 reactions from over 10,000 consumer complaints, including four kinds of seizures, blindness, sexual dysfunction and death.

FDA gives aspartame/NutraSweet/Equal a green light, and then hunts down a compassionate herbalist to destroy his fields of cancer counteractants.

FDA not only breaks the law but ignores it: When I filed a Citizens Petition to Ban Aspartame, the law required FDA to answer me in 180 days. Mine was filed 7 years ago and they refuse to answer. Notice of an imminent health hazard must be answered in ten days. They stonewalled mine, sent certified on October 24, 2007.

Dr. Verrett said: "What can be done to restore to consumers their right to safe food regardless of economic and political interests? . . . Probably the best solution, as some members of Congress have suggested, is to abolish the FDA and start over with a completely new agency free of some of the political pressures. . . . When science and the public interest win out, it is invariably only after the government has been pushed to the wall by consumer advocates and other public pressure."

During the Dietary Supplement Bill era the FDA went wild with raids, even with guns when they called on Dr. Jonathan Wright. Then there came the parade with banners. One sign said, "Dr. Wright made me well. FDA Go to Hell."

Today, is the FDA at least worried that a deadly drug is masquerading as an additive and interacting with drugs? Do they care that there are over millions of cases of drug interactions?

No, the FDA is only concerned about a little root that might eliminate cancer.

Benjamin Rush was once said to make this statement: "Unless we put medical freedoms into the Constitution, the time will come when medicine will organize into an undercover dictatorship... All such laws are un-American and despotic, and have no place in a republic... The Constitution of the republic should make special privilege for medical freedom as well as religious freedom." Today there is some question as to who really made that statement, but there was always a higher authority." Genesis 1:29: And God went on to say: "Here I have given to you all vegetation bearing seed which is on the surface of the whole earth, and every tree on which there is the fruit of a tree bearing seed. To you let it serve as food." No FDA approval required.

Here Is The Eve Geller Cancer Formula:
Eve Geller Memorial Cancer Information;
Herbal Formulas Ideas To Support Cancer Treatment

Chawktau Indian Recipes
[Note: After discussion with an Herbalist who sends out the herbs, these are our best guesses at the botanical names. It would be helpful to have a local botanist verify the exact species names]

LYDIA'S PREPARATION #55 Herbs Needed
1. Common Name(s): Rhubarb Root
   Family: Polygonaceae
   Genus: Rheum
   Species: rhaponticum

2. Common Name(s): Spikenard
    Family: Araliaceae
    Genus: Aralia
    Species: racemosa

3. Common Name(s): Black Snakeroot, Sangrel, Virginia Snakeroot
    Serpentaria, Red River Snakeroot, Texas Snakeroot, Birthwort,
    Sangre Root
    Family: Aristolochiaceae
    Genus: Aristolochia
    Species: serpentaria
    Special Info: SHOULD be harvested on upper part of
    mountain, above 3,300 ft. The higher the better as environment
    conditions change the plant chemistry.

    Use *no more* than 25% extra black snakeroot if harvested at
    lower elevations.

4. Common Name(s): Ladyslipper
    Family: Orchidaceae
    Genus: Cypridium
    Species: pubescens
    Special Info: Endangered species. Please use with discretion.

Instructions
1. Obtain or make powders of the above-mentioned herbs in the
    following amounts:
    a. 14 Oz. Powdered Rhubarb
    b. 12 Oz. Powdered Spikenard
    c. 4 Oz. Powdered Black Snakeroot
    d. 6 Oz. Powdered Ladyslipper

2. Mix the powders thoroughly. This will make a six month's supply of powder.

3. Dosage:
   Adult: 1/2 teaspoon or equivalent amount in #2 capsules after each meal (3 times per day).

   Children: Not recommended.

LYDIAS PREPARATION #99
Herbs & Supplies Needed

1. Common Name(s): Black Cohosh Root, Rattle Root, Squaw Root, Snake Root
   Family: Ranculaceae
   Genus: Cimicifuga
   Species: racemosa

2. Common Name(s): Spikenard
   Family: Araliaceae
   Genus: Aralia
   Species: racemosa

3. Common Name: Wild Cherry Bark, Choke Cherry, Chokeberry
   Family: Rosaceae
   Genus: Prunus
   Species: virginiana

4. Common Name: Mullein Leaf
   Family: Scrophulariaceae
   Genus: Verbascum
   Species: thaspus

5. Common Name(s): Ladyslipper
   Family: Orchidaceae
   Genus: Cypridium
   Species: pubescens
   Special Info: Endangered species. Please use with discretion.

6. Common Name(s): Tincture of Iron, Ferrous Sulfate
   Special Info: Optional. Can purchase from drug store.

WARNING: Do not use iron or ferrous sulfate if you have an iron metabolism disorder which causes excess buildup of iron. For example, primary hemochromatosis affects 3 to 8/1000 persons.

Not part of the original formula, but added by non-Native Americans:
7. Common Name(s): Quinine Sulfate
   Special Info: Preferred, but optional. Requires a prescription today but at one time you could get this at your local drug store.
   The original formula called for the inner bark of a dogwood (green oozer) tree. It contains quinine. At least 10 times more dogwood bark was used than the concentrated quinine sulfate.

   For a readily-obtainable, natural replacement use:
   a. Common Name(s): Cinchona Bark
       Family: Rubiaceae
       Genus: Cinchona
       Species: succirubra
       Special Info: Boil and simmer with other herbs (see below).

8. Common Name(s): Oil of Wintergreen
   Family: Ericaceae
   Genus: Gaultheria
   Species: procumbens
   Special Info: MUST use unrefined, *edible* variety.

Instructions

1. Herbs should be dried, and then cut & sifted, except ladyslipper is powdered.

2. Using a 7 gallon container, place the following in layers, starting from the bottom:
   a. 2 lbs. 3 Oz. Black Cohash
   b. 1 lb. Spikenard
   c. 4 Oz. Cherry Bark
   d. 8 Oz. Mullein Leaf
   e. 4 Oz. Ladyslipper Powder

3. Fill the container 3/4 of the way full of water, bring to a boil then turn to a simmer (not boil) for 8 hours.

4. Remove from heat and let cool for a few hours.

5. Mash juice out of roots.

6. Strain liquid through a cheesecloth or other natural material. Find someone strong who can squeeze out all of the juice.

7. In a quart of natural spring water, mix 1/2 teaspoon of Oil of Wintergreen (edible variety) with 1/4 teaspoon of Quinine Sulfate (preferred) and 12 Oz. of Tincture of Iron or Ferrous Sulfate (optional).

8. Put in bottles and refrigerate when not using. Store unused herbs out of sunlight in dry location. Refrigerate powdered herbs.

9. Dosage:
   One teaspoon immediately before each meal.
   Take formulas for one year.

3

Melanoma
CHEROKEE INDIAN RECIPE
Herbs & Supplies Needed

1. Common Name(s): Sheep Sorrel, Sourgrass, Meadowsorrow, Red Top Sorrel
   Family: Polygonaceae
   Genus: Rumex
   Species: Acetosa
   Special Info: Must be freshly picked --
   no more than two days old.

2. Common Name(s): Pewter Bowl with a *clear* glass cover.

3. Common Name(s): Meat grinder or Heavy Duty blender such as a Vitamix.

Instructions
1. Obtain fresh sheep sorrel by picking it yourself or by 2nd-day air express mail.

2. Put 1 pound through meat grinder. Then put into heavy duty blender until mostly liquefied. Use blender only if necessary, but it must be nearly liquefied when done. Use only a very small amount of spring water in the blender. Just enough to keep the blade spinning and to liquefy the sheep sorrel.

3. Put liquefied sheep sorrel in a pewter bowl outside in the sun and cover with the clear glass cover. It does not need to be completely air tight.

4. Leave it out for five days performing the following tasks:
   a. Take it in during the evening.

b. Wipe condensed liquid from the inside of the cover 3 to 6 times per day using a paper towel.

c. If mold forms during night on the outer skin of the liquid, remove *all* of the mold in the morning before putting it out.

d. Mix every other day

5. After five days it should form a blackish-green, putty-consistency substance. Mix with a little bit of tea tree oil or Vitamin E.

6. It will keep refrigerated for several months. You can freeze it to keep indefinitely.

7. Dosage:
Put on melanoma two to four times every other day using a toothpick. Put on just enough to cover it and do not put on skin surrounding the melanoma. It burns a little bit. You can put a good Band-Aid over it. Just make sure the melanoma stays covered with the substance throughout the day.

Dr. Betty Martini, D.Hum, Founder
Mission Possible International
9270 River Club Parkway
Duluth, Georgia 30097
770 242-2599
www.mpwhi.com, www.dorway.com and www.wnho.net
Aspartame Toxicity Center, www.holisticmed.com/aspartame

Aspartame is a multipotential carcinogen
A Chinese proverb tells us to "Call things by their proper names." The sweetener producers assure us that the chemical aspartame aka: NutraSweet, Spoonful, Equal, E951, Canderel, NutraTaste, etc. is just an additive. To call aspartame what it is: It's an addictive excitoneurotoxic, genetically engineered, carcinogenic drug. It damages the cellular powerhouses, the mitochondria, debilitating cell function. It interacts

with other drugs and vaccines. It often triggers polychemical sensitivity syndrome so greatly intensifying toxic reactions to other chemicals. The body remembers aspartame and ones who have overcome the addiction often experience amplified toxic reactions if they should ingest it again.

The aspartame molecule consists of 3 components, two of which are amino acids that are beneficial nutrients when combined with other amino acids in our foods. However, if isolated aspartic acid, 40% of aspartame, and phenylalanine, 50%, are highly toxic. Some individuals have the condition Phenylketonuria, and have intense toxic reactions to excess phenylalanine. At birth doctors heel-stick infants to analyze their blood to detect this condition. In such cases an excess of this amino acid can be fatal. Excess phenylalanine floods the brain and lowers the seizure threshold and depletes serotonin, the hormone you produce when you've eaten enough. As a result you crave carbohydrates and gain weight... Lowered serotonin triggers psychiatric and behavioral problems. The National Yogurt Assn has petitioned the FDA to allow aspartame in yogurt unlabeled. Any dairy products used today must be organic.

The third part of aspartame, 10%, is a methyl-ester which immediately converts to methyl alcohol, deadly wood alcohol, and methanol. An ounce of this poison can blind or kill an adult. The methyl alcohol next converts to embalming fluid, formaldehyde, then into formic acid, fire ant venom. The whole aspartame molecule breaks down to diketopiperazine, a brain tumor agent.

The bouquet of a half dozen virulent poisons in aspartame is cumulative, and eventually eradicates good health in the same manner as regularly ingesting micro doses of arsenic or plutonium will certainly destroy you. In 1995 the FDA listed 92 symptoms of aspartame poisoning from over 10,000 volunteered consumer complaints. The list included 4 types of seizures, blindness, headaches, sexual dysfunction and death. Most were neurological complaints, since the chemical is neurotoxic. The results are diverse and dispersed all over the body. Some of us remember when there were no constant bombardments on TV of sexual potency restorers; Viagra et al. Aspartame destroys a man's ability and takes away a woman's desire, robbing marriage of a sacred delight.

We have thousands of letters from victims who have been delivered from the devastations of this deadly concoction.

If people saw how aspartame is made they wouldn't use it. Bill Deagle, M.D. said: "Most people when asked how Aspartame is made do not have the first step of understanding. While an E.R. doctor and primary care physician in Augusta, GA in 1987 and 1988, I was told a number of interesting facts about the adjacent Aspartame factory. Bacteria with genes inserted generate a sludge which is centrifuged to remove the aspartame and many hundreds of contaminant organic and amino acids are present. We were told not to report illness or worker's compensation issues for fear of being fired by the hospital, now the Augusta Regional Medical Center. Many of their employees presented with psychiatric, neuropathy conditions, chronic fatigue and organic cases of loss of cognitive function. This powder from the dried sludge was then transported for packaging in factories elsewhere in the US, before sale as Equal and now the myriad of names of this neurotoxin."

It was known from the beginning that aspartame is a carcinogen and absolutely against the law. FDA's own toxicologist, Dr. Adrian Gross, told Congress at least one of Searle's studies "has established beyond any reasonable doubt that aspartame is capable of inducing brain tumors in experimental animals and that this predisposition of it is of extremely high significance. ... In view of these indications that the cancer causing potential of aspartame is a matter that had been established way beyond any reasonable doubt, one can ask: What is the reason for the apparent refusal by the FDA to invoke for this food additive the so-called Delaney Amendment to the Food, Drug and Cosmetic Act?"

The Delaney Amendment makes it illegal to allow any residues of cancer causing chemicals in foods. In his concluding testimony Gross asked, "Given the cancer causing potential of aspartame how would the FDA justify its position that it views a certain amount of aspartame as constituting an allowable daily intake or 'safe' level of it? Is that position in effect not equivalent to setting a 'tolerance' for this food additive and thus a violation of that law? And if the FDA itself elects to violate the law, who is left to protect the health of the public?" Congressional Record

SID835:131 (August 1,1985) In original studies aspartame triggered not only brain tumors but mammary, uterine, ovarian, testicular, pancreatic and thyroid tumors.

In 1996, Ralph Walton, M.D., did research with scientific peer reviews and showed that 92% of independent studies showed the problems aspartame cause. Then in 2005 and 2007 Dr. Morando Soffritti, Ramazzini Institute in Italy, published two monumental studies.

In 2005 he completed three years of impeccable research using 1,800 Sprague-Dawley rats (100-150/per sex/per group). To simulate varying human intake, aspartame was added to the standard rat diet in quantities of 5000, 2500, 100, 500, 20, 4, and 0 milligrams per kilogram of body weight. Treatment of the animals began when they were 8 weeks old, and continued until spontaneous death. The results were dynamic: APM causes a statistically significant, dose-related increase of lymphomas/leukemias and malignant tumors of the renal pelvis in females and malignant tumors of peripheral nerves in males. These results demonstrate for the first time that APM is a carcinogenic agent, capable of inducing malignancies at various dose levels, including those lower than the current acceptable daily intake (ADI) for humans (50 mg/kg of body weight in the US, 40 mg/kg of body weight in the EU).

Doctor Soffritti's second ERF study in 2007 was conducted on 400 Sprague-Dawley rats in much smaller doses to simulate daily human intake. It was added to their diet in quantities of 100, 20, and zero mg/Kg of body weight. Treatment of the animals began on the 12th day of fetal life until natural death. The results of the second study show an increased incidence of lymphomas/leukemias in female rats with respect to the first study. Moreover, the study shows that when lifespan exposure to APM begins during fetal life, the age at which lymphomas/leukemias develop in females is anticipated. For the first time, a statistically significant increase in mammary cancers in females was also observed in the second study. The results of this transplacental carcinogenicity bioassay not only confirm, but also reinforce the first experimental demonstration of APMs multipotential carcinogenicity.

On April 23, 2007, Dr. Soffritti received the Irving J. Selikoff Award for his outstanding contributions to the identification of environmental and industrial carcinogens and his promotion of independent scientific research. It has only been received twice before in history.

Dr. James Bowen points out that "aspartame is a known destroyer of DNA. The mitochondrial DNA (MtDNA) is especially damaged, yielding the present epidemic of diseases aspartame consuming mothers pass on to future generations. Aspartame also directly damages the mitochondria, thus having a 'double whammy' effect on mitochondrial function! The summation of these many known severe toxicities and its immune, genetic, mitochondrial, and metabolic damages, show that aspartame will not only cause many diseases, which the FDA and CDC have already noted but it has pathways of approach to interact adversely with every conceivable pharmaceutical."

According to the second Ramazzini Study if a pregnant women uses aspartame and the baby survives since aspartame triggers birth defects and mental retardation the child can grow up and have cancer.

The European Food Safety Authority with people on its committee connected to the aspartame business attempted to rebut the Ramazzini Studies and blamed the rat deaths on "respiratory disease." They know full well respiratory disease is the dying process. Professionals had a big laugh over that. Every burglar has an alibi!

Dr. Morando Soffritti said: "In examining the raw data of our study, the EFSA (2006) observed a high incidence of chronic pulmonary inflammation in males and females in both treated groups and in the control group. Based on this observation, it was concluded that "the increased incidence of lymphomas/leukemias reported in treated rats was unrelated to aspartame, given the high background incidence of chronic inflammatory changes in the lungs . . ." In my opinion, this conclusion is bizarre for the following reasons:

First, the EFSA (2006) overlooked the fact that the study was conducted until the natural death of the rodents. It is well known that infectious pathologies are part of the natural dying process in both rodents and humans.

Second, if the statistically significant increased incidence of lymphomas/leukemias observed were indeed caused by an infected colony, one would expect to observe an increased incidence of lymphomas/leukemias not only in females but also in males. The EFSA (2006) did not comment on this discrepancy in their logic.

Finally Dr. Herman Koeter of EFSA fessed up and admitted that commercial pressure controlled them with these words in his article *EU's Food Agency Battles Attempts to Hijack Science:* "Science and politics make poor bedfellows. Just ask Herman Koeter, deputy executive director at the European Food Safety Authority (EFSA) which has felt the push and pull of national politics ever since the agency began operating four years ago."

Koeter described the various political pressures EFSA faces as it strives to maintain a firm line between its independent scientific research and the mire of EU politics. Hot decisions that had political repercussions included... *A Review of a Controversial Aspartame Study.*

"Pressure comes from the European Commission, national legislators, regulatory agencies and industry to tone down or beef up results. Sometimes the pressure comes in the form of a push for a firm opinion on controversial subjects, when science is unable to yield a clear answer," Koeter said. Now Dr. Koeter is no longer with EFSA but at least before he left he told the world the truth.

Attorney James Turner, author of "The Chemical Feast: The Nader Report on Food Protection at the FDA," was the consumer attorney who with neuroscientist Dr. John Olney, legally fought the approval of aspartame from 1973 until 1985. He has reviewed with disappointment the European Food Safety Authority panel's original and amended conclusions on the second Ramazzini Study.

Mr. Turner states:

It is impossible to say that Aspartame is not a carcinogen. This conclusion of the 1980 FDA Public Board of Inquiry remains true today. FDA's own scientist Dr. Adrian Gross, who worked on the FDA investigative team that revealed dozens of legal volition in the Aspartame's studies conducted by Searle Drug Company, acknowledged that aspartame violated the Delaney Amendment because of this.

The approval of aspartame was the most contested in FDA history. The sweetener was not approved on scientific grounds but through strong political and financial pressure and through the political chicanery of Donald Rumsfeld who ran the company making aspartame. The European Food Safety Authority argues that the high incidence of cancerous tumors that occurred in the Ramazzini studies are caused by something other than aspartame. However there were high incidences of cancerous tumors in studies provided to support aspartame's FDA approval.

There was also a significant increase in human cancerous tumors like those in animals in the first year of aspartame's use in diet sodas. The record is too damning for any informed individual to risk their own health by consuming aspartame. Aspartame should never have been approved and actions to ban it started soon after approval as victims suffered from seizures, MS, blindness, cancer and death. The FDA listed 92 reactions attributed to this poison.

When I testified before Congress in 1987, I stated that 'just because a substance reaches the market it should not be treated as sacrosanct. It must be recognized that over time a substance that we know harms people will continue to harm people. .. If the standard of food safety is that a substance that only harms some people, but not all people is going to be allowed on the market, then special policies should be adopted to protect those at risk.' This was never done.

Since approval, victims of aspartame continue to develop neurodegenerative disease, suffer diabetes, drug interactions, obesity, heart disease and loss of vision. Never has the public been warned that it triggers birth defects, a catastrophe the eminent Dr. Louis Elsas warned Congress about. In fact the average consumer of aspartame is not aware that the European Food Safety Authority says that an acceptable daily intake (ADI) of aspartame is 40 milligrams/kilogram of body weight about the amount in a six pact of diet soda for a 10 year old boy. Nor do they know how to tell if that amount is being exceeded by intake of the more than 5000 food and drug products currently sweetened with aspartame.

Enough from EFSA! The entire aspartame fiasco is documented. The only responsible thing to do is ban it. And if they refuse to ban it, then it should carry heavy warnings including a statement of the ADI and the amount of aspartame in every product. The Ramazzini Study has confirmed twice what the FDA knew from the beginning. To loose upon an entire unwarned continent a chemical that destroys the fetus, triggers mental illness and cancer, and sickens millions without a word of warning is corrupt and depraved. EFSA is responsible to prevent such depredations not simply protect the greedy pockets of poison producers.

Mr. Turner tells the story of aspartame approval in
Sweet Misery: A Poisoned World.
Here is that clip: http://www.soundandfury.tv/pages/rumsfeld.html
Russell Blaylock, M.D. Neurosurgeon: Author: *Excitotoxins: the Taste That Kills* and *Natural Strategies for Cancer Patients* commenting on both Ramazzini studies, said: "My review of the first Ramazzini Study concluded that the study was one of the best designed, comprehensive and conclusive studies done to date on the multipotential carcinogenic danger of aspartame. This second study is even more conclusive, in that it shows a dose-dependent statistically significant increase in lymphomas/leukemia in both male and female rats exposed to aspartame. These two cancers are the fastest growing cancers in

people under age 30.

Also, of major concern is their finding of statistically significant increases in breast cancer in animals exposed to aspartame. With newer studies clearly indicating that toxic exposures during fetal development can dramatically increase the cancer risk of the offspring, this study takes on a very important meaning to all pregnant women consuming aspartame products. Likewise, small children are at considerable risk of the later development of these highly fatal cancers. It should be appreciated that the doses used in these studies fall within the range of doses seen in everyday users of aspartame. This study, along with the first study, should convince any reasonable scientific mind, as well as the public, that this product should be removed from the market. http://www.russellblaylockmd.com

The nation of Romania banned aspartame in the early 1990's because it caused cancer. EFSA must think aspartame only causes cancer in Romania, not the rest of the world.

H. J. Roberts, M.D., FACP, Palm Beach Institute for Medical Research, who authored the 1,000 page medical text, *Aspartame Disease: An Ignored Epidemic*, also reviewed EFSA's deceitful report. He said, "The ongoing attempts to ridicule clinical, epidemiologic and experimental studies warning of probable carcinogenic effects of aspartame products are both dubious and retrogressive—particularly in the case of brain tumors, breast cancer and leukemia/lymphoma. I have reviewed the evidence in my corporate-neutral publications, and in submissions to the legislatures of several states seeking to ban the products and the European Food Safety Authority. This is not an academic consideration when over half the population has been consuming these products. Moreover, I disagree with the AFC Panel that there is no reason to revise the ADI for aspartame of 40 mg/kg bw... as detailed in my texts. www.sunsentpress.com.

EFSA's mammary tumor excuse is preposterous. It was always known aspartame triggers mammary tumors. Alex Constantine, who wrote

NutraPoison, discussed how aspartame was listed with the Pentagon in an inventory of prospective biochemical warfare weapons submitted to Congress said:

> G. D. Searle (original manufacturer) submitted a battery of cancer-test results, titled the Willigan Report, which contained a statistical table that wrongly excluded four malignant, aspartame-related mammary tumors detected by Dr. Willigan and incorporated in his initial data. Somehow, the malignancies were made to appear benign. Searle dismissed the misrepresentation as a computer error, claiming that the unfavorable mammary malignancy data were innocently omitted from the summary table four separate times by three different individuals.

Dr. Ken Stoller declared: "EFSA's position on aspartame is a testament to the power of corporations to influence, compromise and corrupt the safety nets that have been put into place to protect the public."

Everything on aspartame is a matter of public record and the reports listed on web sites such as www.mpwhi.com, www.dorway.com, www.wnho.net and www.holisticmed.com/aspartame Dr. Maria Alemany, who did the Trocho Study showing that the formaldehyde converted from the free methyl alcohol embalms living tissue told me when I consulted him in Barcelona: "Betty, aspartame will kill 200 million."

Many times this poison is hidden in things that say artificial and natural flavors so you have to avoid processed foods. For 18 years I've taken the case histories of the sick and dying and it's hard when you hear a young girl with a head full of aspartame brain tumors cry: "I want to live, I want to live, I want to live."

Aspartame causes everything from MS, lupus, blindness and seizures to sudden cardiac death. Do not use it - your life depends on it. There have been three congressional hearings and efforts to ban it ever since it was marketed due to the political chicanery of Donald Rumsfeld who was CEO of Searle to get it approved. The FDA had revoked the petition for approval. However, if you don't buy it they can't sell it! Also do not use Splenda, a chlorocarbon poison. "Just Like Sugar" is a safe sweetener usually sold in Whole Foods. It's just chicory, orange peel, Vitamin C and Calcium.

"Deliver those who are being taken away to death; and those staggering to the slaughter, O may you hold them back. In case you should say: 'Look! We did not know of this,' will not he himself that is making an estimate of hearts discern it, and he himself that is observing your soul know and certainly pay back to earthling man according to his activity" (Proverbs 24: 11, 12).

The Lethal Science of Splenda:
http://www.wnho.net/splenda_chlorocarbon.htm

Studies have shown that sucralose can:
- Cause the thymus to shrink by as much as 40% (the thymus is your immune powerhouse—it produces T cells)
- Cause enlargement of the liver and kidneys
- Reduce growth rate as much as 20%
- Cause enlargement of the large bowel area
- Reduce the amount of good bacteria in the intestines by 50%
- Increase the pH level in the intestines (a high risk factor for colon cancer)
- Contribute to weight gain
- Cause aborted pregnancy low fetal body weight
- Reduce red blood cell count

Particular warning to diabetics: Researchers found that diabetic patients using sucralose showed a statistically significant increase in glycosylated hemoglobin, a marker that is used to assess glycemic control in diabetic patients. According to the FDA, "increases in glycosolation in hemoglobin imply lessening of control of diabetes."

For the most complete and profound information on these issues visit my friend Dr. Betty Martini's websites:

www.mpwhi.com
www.dorway.com
www.wnho.net

Dr. Betty Martini, D.Hum, Founder
Mission Possible International
9270 River Club Parkway
Duluth, Georgia 30097
770 242-2599

Mission Possible International is a global volunteer force in the US and 40 nations warning the world of aspartame.

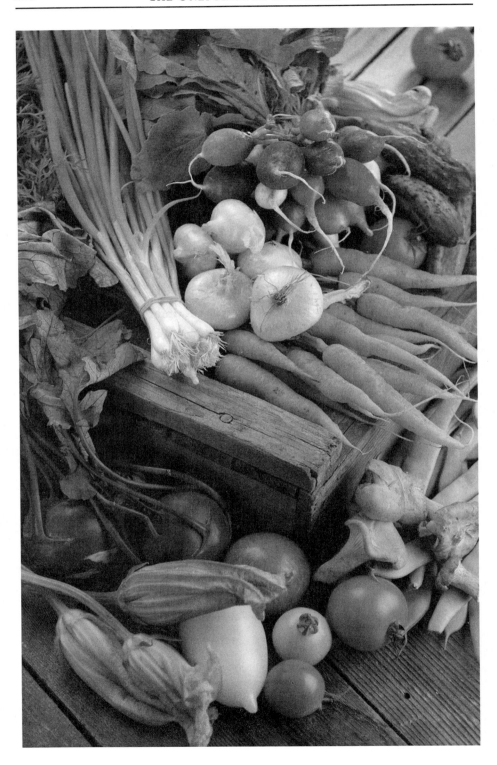

DIET FOR CANCER PATIENTS

Paul Nison

"There is a Time to Every Purpose Under the Heaven."

—Ecclesiastes 3:1

Article written by Paul Nison, Author/Speaker and Raw Food Gourmet Chef www.PaulNison.com

Official website of author Paul Nison: www.RawLife.com - Health E-store for all your health needs

Can diet heal cancer?

If you ask most doctors today, nothing can "heal" cancer. They will try to cut it out, burn it and kill it. Sometimes they have success in temporally slowing down the inevitable. The reason why they will never have a cure is because as long as the root cause is not removed, the problem will always be there.

Stress is a major root cause of cancer and must be reduced and eliminated. Removing stress from your life allows the body to do what it was designed to do; be healthy and disease free.

Where does diet come into play? Identifying stressful areas in your life is the first step toward reclaiming your health. Lack of enjoyment for life, money issues, worry and fear build stress, but the most common stress on the body is eating and abusing harmful foods.

Abusing foods is the most common stress to the body. People consume foods that were never meant to be in our body, they eat foods in amounts that their body can't manage, and they eat at times they shouldn't be eating.

Before viewing my diet suggestions, please understand that health begins with what you eliminate from your diet, not with what you add. The first step in recovery and healing is to remove the problem foods from your diet. Then you can replace them with the healthy food you should have been eating from the beginning.

Cancer can only come alive and grow in a body that is lacking oxygen. The average person today, especially someone with cancer, is walking around with a serious case of insufficient oxygen. The following tips are musts if you are serious about overcoming cancer.

First we will discuss what we should eliminate from our diet.

Processed foods

Eating highly processed foods prevents the body from receiving oxygen. Every bite taken from foods that come in a bag, container, box, can, bottle or bag is contributing to cancer. I tell everyone to be wary of eating these foods, especially foods without an expiration date. Healthy food is supposed to spoil after a few weeks, even a month. But if it lasts much longer, be wary. It's most likely very processed with many chemicals and other drugs to prolong the shelf life of the food while shortening the life of your body.

New Foods

If it wasn't food one hundred years ago, don't consider it food today. New foods also have new drugs and chemicals in them in amounts that are harmful to the body. Big business has created many of these foods because they care more about your wallet than your health.

Dead Foods

If you put a food in the ground and it doesn't grow, don't put it in your body. Foods that have their enzymes in them are known as live foods because they produce and support life. You can put the seeds of these foods into the ground and you will have a tree or plant growing. Foods that lack enzymes are known as dead foods and support death.

I am a teacher at the world's foremost health institute that specializes in healing people with cancer: Hippocrates Health Institute (HHI) in West Palm Beach, Florida. (I highly suggest to everyone with a cancer diagnosis or other health challenges to go there. Mention my name for a discount). At HHI, they discovered key essentials to help the body heal itself of cancer. Two of the most common suggestions are to eat live foods with their enzymes intact, and include a highly-green, chlorophyll-rich diet. Keep in mind that cooking destroys all enzymes in foods and a person trying to heal from cancer should consume a 100% raw, live-food diet.

Sugars

The directors of HHI recommend that all people healing cancer should avoid all sugars, even sugars found in fruits. Most people are aware that processed sugars are not healthful, but knowledge is lacking in regards to "natural" sugars, such as those found in fruits.

Regardless of the type of sugar consumed, too much sugar can cause problems. It leads to fermentation in the body that feeds and promotes yeast growth and negative bacteria. Overeating sugary foods causes constipation and gas, and this gas can back up into the bloodstream. This is where most diseases originate—from candida to cancer and everything in between. If you want to be healthy, you must learn to cut back on sugary and starchy foods.

One last tip on things to avoid: If food has to go through the car window, it definitely shouldn't be in your body.

Three things to consume if you want to overcome cancer

1. Eat high quality food

If you have cancer you must treat your body the best way possible. This means only consuming food raw, ripe, fresh organic and live. Once you are healed, you can cut back to 80% of your foods meeting this criteria, but 100% is still best.

The main part of your diet should be raw vegetables and sprouts, such as leafy green vegetables, wheatgrass, algae, sea vegetables, and sunflower sprouts. The reason these green foods are so beneficial for the body is that they contain chlorophyll—the blood of plants.

Chlorophyll is the pigment that gives trees, grasses, and leafy plants their characteristic, green color. More importantly, chlorophyll enables plants to convert the sun's energy into nutrients that can be utilized by living organisms. Chlorophyll is similar to hemoglobin in human blood. Chlorophyll-rich, plant juices supply rich, soil-based minerals, vitamins, and chlorophyll proteins to our diet, plus it contains oxygen.

Foods high in chlorophyll include wheatgrass, which is used at health spas around the world to treat cancer and other deadly diseases, and sea algae which is available in several edible forms.

The foods you should emphasize in your diet are fresh vegetables (green vegetables are best but others are also helpful), non-sweet fruits such as cucumbers, zucchini, bell peppers and squash. For example, cucumbers, zucchini, bell peppers and squash are technically considered fruits because they have seeds. Because they are non-sweet fruits, they are delicious additions to the diet.

Also there should be nuts and seeds in your diet. Soaking nuts and seeds for 6 to 12 hours releases enzymes which allows for easier digestion. It's very easy to consume too many nuts, so be careful.

Whole grains and legumes can be eaten but it's best to eat grains that have been sprouted first, so they are easier to digest. The least healthful grains are rye, spelt, basmati rice, white rice, wheat, barley, and corn. The most healthful grains are: millet, quinoa, amaranth, teff, buckwheat (hulled).

Of all the foods mentioned that are okay to consume, sea vegetables and sprouts are the most beneficial. These are the highest quality land and sea vegetation for our nutrients. Some popular sea vegetables are alaria, arame, dulse, hijiki and nori.

Sprouted food is any type of seed, nut, grain, or bean that has been soaked in water, exposed to air and indirect sunlight, and if rinsed daily, has started to form a new plant, beginning with a sprout. Some examples include: almond sprouts, buckwheat sprouts, sunflower sprouts and mung bean sprouts. Sprouted foods are one of the highest forms of food you can put into your body. They are very helpful for the building of new cells, and provide the cells with oxygen. Green sprouts are very high in chlorophyll.

2. Eat at the right times

I just wrote a new book called *The Daylight Diet* (the book can be purchased at www.rawlife.com.) The point of the book is to understand that we have been designed to be on schedule if we want to be healthy!

We have all the tools we need and all the intelligence to know the best schedule for us to enjoy a healthy, long, satisfying life. Of the many ideas and concepts regarding nutrition and what foods are most nutritious for the human body, the majority of people have not taken into consideration the times of eating for best digestion.

We have been designed to eat certain foods, and at certain times of the day. Just as water in your gas tank will harm the car, bad foods will harm your body. A car is made to run on certain fuel and so is our body. However, no matter what time of the day you put gas in your gas tank, it won't make a difference. The time you put fuel in your body, however, does make a big difference.

It was our Creator who first separated the salt water from the fresh, made dry land, and planted a garden. He made animals and fish before making even one human being. He provided what we needed before He even created us. If He designed our body and He knows every single hair on our heads, I'm sure he knows what we should eat and when we should eat it.

He created the heavens and the earth, including humans, food, sun, and the moon. The sun and the moon set the schedule we have been designed to follow. The information I share in this book can lead to a healthy life only if we stop watching man's calendar and clock and base our time by the sun and the moon each day.

When the sun is up, feel free to eat; when it is down, stop. I can't make this advice any simpler than that! Eat your meals as long as the sun is up and it is light outside. But when it is dark and the moon is rising, your meals should end for the day. This is the number one rule of the Daylight Diet. If you stick to this important principle, you will see excellent results in your health, energy, sleep—your whole being—because this is how we have been designed to eat. Nighttime is for resting and sleeping.

Don't eat late in the day. You will get better sleep, have better digestion, slow down the aging process, have more energy, and feel wonderful. Just stop eating late in the day—especially when it's dark outside—and experience for yourself the great results.

Practicing temperance in eating will rejuvenate your whole body and rid you of most health problems. Your goal should be to reduce the number of meals you consume and reduce the amount of food in those meals, while making sure you are consuming the highest quality food.

The real key to success is to avoid eating at nighttime, and go to sleep on an empty stomach. Food shouldn't be a daily struggle. I can attest that it may not be easy at first, but to be truly successful, you will have to change your thinking along with your diet.

3. Eat the right way

When eating, being in a relaxed environment is very important. It's never healthy to eat when stressed no matter how good the food is. In addition, along with the amount of food, number of meals, quality of food, and times you eat that all affect digestion; there is more that needs to be done to keep your body healthy.

After we swallow, the food we've eaten is more or less out of our control. Before that, though, we have total control: Proper mastication and food combining can prevent many digestive problems.

Digestion begins in the mouth. Saliva contains an enzyme that helps break down the food and jumpstarts digestion. Chewing helps the body more readily extract the nutrients from the food and cuts down on the work the digestive system has to do. The less work the digestive tract has to do; the more efficiently it will do its job. When we don't chew our food well, it can ferment in our digestive system. The more food is chewed, the easier it is to digest, and the healthier it will be for the body. Even raw foods can cause problems if they're not properly chewed.

Food combining

The types of food we eat together, called food combining, play a big role in good digestion. Eating the wrong foods together or in the wrong order can sap our energy and cause fermenting and putrefaction in the digestive system.

Food combining allows for easier digestion and minimal digestive conflicts. It works like this: Every food takes a certain amount of time to digest. Eating similar foods with similar digestive times helps the body digest meals more easily; these foods are said to combine well. For example, watermelon takes about one hour to digest; almonds may take up to five hours. In view of this, eating watermelon and almonds at the same meal is not a good idea, so it's known as a poor combination. Eating too many meals like this may cause constipation, bloating, and gas, which may lead to more serious issues.

Final Thought

The human body is amazing when we treat it the way we're supposed to. We were designed to eat certain types of foods—raw, fresh, organic fruits, vegetables, nuts, and seeds—to keep our digestive systems moving and clean. Good health comes only when we have good digestion, and that good digestion only results when we eat properly and healthfully.

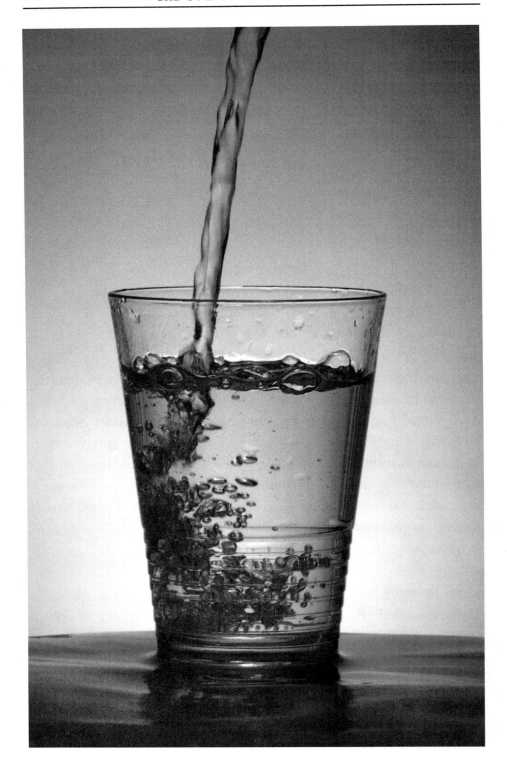

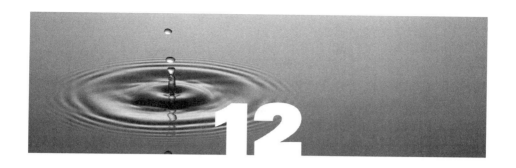

WATER: THE UNIVERSAL ELEMENT OF LIFE AND OF DEATH

FRED VAN LIEW

Contributed by Fred Van Liew
The world knows Fred as The Water Doctor
www.ewater.com www.trinisol.com

First, we start with some words of caution: pH in water does not necessarily determine pH in the body. You are not necessarily looking for alkaline or oxygen rich water. Both can be desirable under the right conditions; however the presence of either does not mean they will be utilized effectively. A small amount of any acid in pure water will register the water as acid; however the lack of any real substance will fail to acidify the body. This is often the case of slightly acid reverse osmosis water. Alkalize your body with proper nourishment, not water. You can artificially alkalize your body with ionizers and pH drops of all kinds, as well as coral calcium. Some of these may jam your kidneys, clog your lymphatics and make you feel good while you continue to decline in health. This is not healing. The purity, energies and structure of water can be far more important factors to your health restoration and maintenance, both short term and long term.

A wise man, when asked what type of water purifier or filter to use, answered in this manner: "If you ask Fred Van Liew, he is going to say reverse osmosis is the best way to go. If you ask WaterWise, they are going to say distilled is the only way to go. If you ask MultiPure, they are going to say carbon block is the only way to go. He then said what they all agree on, however, is that you absolutely do not drink the tap water. Do your homework and choose. Just do not drink untreated tap water." That man was my very close friend Kevin Trudeau. He has practiced what he teaches for many years and is the real deal. I recommend you listen to him often on KTRADIONETWORK.com and read his books if you want to know what is really going on in health and politics. His advice on water is still true and is a good starting point for any discussion.

Flouride is more toxic than lead

There is a poison commonly added to water that is more toxic than lead and only slightly less toxic than arsenic. That poison is fluoride. Whether in its sodium fluoride form, primarily a by-product of aluminum and metal smelting, or the more commonly used highly acidic hydrofluorosilicic liquid washdown from SuperPhosphate smokestacks, this poison disrupts all seven collagen proteins in the body. Research consistently has shown fluoride in water forms some of the rarest cancers known. It is one of the most abundant substances on the planet; it is highly toxic to the body when ingested, unless it has been digested first by plants.

Fluoride is almost impossible to remove except by distillation or reverse osmosis. Some filter media like activated alumina can reduce sodium fluoride by up to 50%, however it is far less effective with the more commonly used hydrofluorosilicic acid form of Fluoride. Bone Char will reduce either form of fluoride, however the operative term is only reduce, and often not significantly. Other substances and metals in the water can dramatically change removal characteristics.

Our drinking water is being used as the disposal system of an exceptionally toxic poison by government and industry to avoid enormous waste disposal costs. All this comes at the cost of our children's health.

When added to the nearly 40 some odd toxin loaded vaccinations a child now receives by the time they are seven year old, this creates a health nightmare for the body. Vaccine components like Mercury, aluminum, live and dead viral elements, formaldehyde, and just about any form of filth they can find to place in these vaccines continue to be implicated in the compromise of our immune systems and to produce death. Adjuvants like Squaline have been shown to produce horrible neurological disorders and increase the effect of good and questionable substances in unproven vaccines. The combination of fluoride poison and vaccine poison accumulating and combining like a chemistry set makes you wonder how even this miraculous body can survive….OR IS IT SURVIVING?

We are finding medical wastes in our processed drinking water. Chlorine added to our drinking water combines with pesticides, medical wastes, and other chemicals to produce chlorinated by-products (CBP's). Chlorine reacts with organic matter to form THM's or TriHaloMethanes. All of these are either cancer causing, tumorogenic, or teratogenic, (interfering with the growth of an embryo).

We have heavy metals, the most common being lead, however cadmium and Zinc are common, as is copper leaching from pipes, and aluminum, especially in wells. East Texas wells were found to have high levels of Aluminum. Aluminum is very interesting in that it masks all kinds of problems, including preventing the elimination of acid water conditions. It also is difficult to remove with a filter. Arsenic is problematic in different parts of the country. We've had babies being born with all kinds of health challenges in Grand Prairie, Texas two decades ago because of the public wells contaminated with heavy metals and high fluoride. This nearly cost my newly born son his life, even after going through the largest carbon block made at the time. You see, I did my homework, chose the best filter recommended. I found too late that

I had been lied to by both the written research and by the manufacturers. You see, Filter manufacturers will tell you what their filters will do, however they don't tell you what they won't do. We had women in our Church with distended stomachs and hair falling out from what was later believed to be the water from those wells in Grand Prairie, which thankfully are now all shut down. Babies were born with all kinds of health challenges, much like my son, and like my son there were many dental challenges in those early developmental months and years. Our friend's child, born a few miles away shortly after my son, had his teeth turn to near powder shortly after they finally came in. These are some of the horror stories that drove me into water purification full time.

Nitrates and other toxins in water

Nitrates are another example of a serious challenge when found in water. A young couple with small children, were renting a house with a well that contained about 30 ppm Nitrates. When they called they were told what they should do to correct the problem. You should not even bathe in those levels of Nitrates. They procrastinated for over a year, and only called when a brain tumor had developed in one of their children. This tragedy was entirely preventable had they not failed to take immediate remedial action.

Hard water is another common challenge in many parts of the country. Seven grains is considered hard and water that is less than fifteen Grains hardness, or about 250 ppm calcium hardness, should consider alternatives to water softening. Water softening uses salts of one type or another that may compromise our health and the environment. We have successfully treated water that was over 180 grains hardness, and that doctor told us in no uncertain terms that you did not have to be Jesus Christ to walk on his well water. A simple request to your water company will get you a current comprehensive analysis of your water, which they are required by law now to provide or face stiff penalties.

Other poisons and toxins, like dioxin, are not even tested, as they are often found in water and the municipalities simply cannot afford to remove them. Some are exceptionally toxic, with only small amounts able to pose serious health risks.

These are just a few of the many challenges we face, and our source waters keep changing as well. Cities and towns blend waters from different sources to keep testing within parameters, which means you really don't always know day to day what you are going to get from your faucet or your shower.

Bathing and showering exposes you to toxins and poisons

Did you know that bathing or showering exposes you to more water born toxins and poisons than drinking that same water? You climb into a hot shower, pull the curtain shut or close the door, allowing the vapors to concentrate like in a gas chamber. Your skin cells are screaming for help, trying to close your pores, while your energy is being sapped from you body. Some of you even sing! You get out thinking you are relaxed, while in reality you are exhausted. You end up with dry skin and unruly hair, and none the wise for it. When you use an effective shower filter that takes out more than just the chlorine, you get instant response from a grateful body. You climb out refreshed rather than exhausted. You sleep better and you work better. Your hair becomes consistently softer and more elegant, while the skin literally loses those large pores around the nose and gets baby skin soft. Rashes and itching can disappear just from a shower using an effective filter. A whole home filtration system is even better, though not a water softener without filtration. Water softeners do not remove chlorine or chemicals, or may do so for a very short time. They actually can increase your exposure to the health destroying chemicals while increasing the negative effects of the chemicals.

Testing as they relate to water purification choices can be deceptive. In one research experiment, they took cadmium and added it to softened water and to water that was hard (mostly due to calcium). The rats that drank the soft water with cadmium got hyperactive, while those that drank the hard water with cadmium did not get so hyperactive. Their conclusion was that hard water was better for you than soft water. Not true. Hard water WITH CADMIUM IS BETTER for you than soft water with cadmium. Watch out for "Research." When ewater would seek testing for filters, the lab would always ask what results I would like. They were surprised when I told them real results from real testing. You see, they can set up the parameters of a test to make a filter look much better than it is. Slow flow of water or a very small amount of water, may allow certain contaminants to be temporarily held back until more water is passed through the filter. Even a carbon filter will show fluoride reduction with this gimmick. This kind of soured us on a lot of testing claims, although testing can be an indication of actual results.

My own son was poisoned with fluoride, metals and high dissolved solids flowing right through a huge carbon block selected after much research. The fact that the limitations of the carbon block technology were not revealed in the research. This set in motion a quest to find out what every type of water filter or filtration technology would do and what they would not do.

Selecting your course of action.

The first step is to purify or at least filter the water. There are then imprints and memories of the poisons removed that may remain in the water. These must be erased, or you may react, as my own son did, to the memory of fluoride or another substance inprint. You would see his complexion turn sallow and his eye sockets get sunken, just from the memory of fluoride in the water. Years ago we erased these memories with a homeopathic water catalyst and a fractionally distilled aloe vera juice.

1. At the top of my list would be a quality reverse osmosis system. Reverse osmosis will retain many of the properties of the water entering the system, including energies and structure. Unfortunately, these often are absent in the water entering our homes.

2. Next best would be distillation. Distilled is dead water, void of energy and oxygen. It is aggressively trying to fill the voids between its water molecules, as Dr. M.T. Morter writes in his college text "Correlative Urinalysis."

3. Next, a Fluoride reducing filter pitcher using a special media that actually reduces fluoride by up to 65%. This is highly unusual removal for a non reverse osmosis or distillation process. It is the only filter at this time that I know reduces all forms of fluoride substantially.

4. Carbon Block with lead removal capability. Does not remove fluoride, sulfates, nitrates, arsenic, aluminum, phosphates, salts, detergents, metallic and dead dirt minerals, nor virus. Care must be exercised in its use.

5. KDF/Carbon combination. Same limitations as Carbon block, however KDF (Zinc/Copper composite), sometimes referred to as redox media, increased the life of the carbon and reduces lead and copper. It also adds some bacteriostatic properties to the filter.

6. Almost never use just granular carbon alone for drinking water, as it allows too many contaminants and biological activity to pass through.

7. Bone char was used in some drinking water filters. It is charcoal made from cow bones, the best being cow bones from India fired in Scotland. Unfortunately, with what I know now, I would not recommend this for ongoing drinking. These are best used in whole home systems for bathing and showering or brushing teeth.

8. Specialty filters for lead removal, arsenic, fluoride, etc. may be added when necessary.

9. Deionizing cartridges (not good for drinking water) make water very pure however far too aggressive for use in the body.

10. Ozone is for biological purification only with moderate breakdown of some chemicals. Not recommended for ongoing drinking water in most applications and leaves a taste to the water as well.

It can get a little awkward if you keep adding multiple filters. It makes more sense to use a reverse osmosis system with its quality membrane combined with sediment, carbon and carbon block technology to remove most all challenges known and unknown. The exception is the imprinting and revitalizing. These must be dealt with separately.

So, after you purify, you want to energize, structure and harmonically revitalize your water for optimal support of your cellular function and communication. So we must erase the negative memory in water, then hexagonally structure the water, and increase or replace the lost life supporting natural harmonic energies water is supposed to inherently provide.

Once you have created reverse osmosis or distilled water, you want to place your water into an appliance like the Vitalizer Plus, while making sure it has the harmonizing properties found in eCrystal technology added inside the VitalizerPlus.

Both distillation and Reverse osmosis should be used with a Vitalizer Plus machine and an eCrystal with BioEnergies. Another option is to use harmonizing water catalysts such as QuantaWater, Perfect Balance or Harmony drops as good examples. The VitalizerPlus replicates nature, and the eCrystal brings back the high level harmonics that take the water from a solid 65% hydration after the water is spun in the Vitalizer Plus alone and brings it up to 85-100% intra-cellular hydration.

What about Acid/Alkaline ionizers?

Acid/Alkaline Ionizers, if used with Reverse osmosis, can add an abundance of electrons. Most of these units are not recommended with their carbon only filtration, as it does not remove fluoride or many harmful poisons in the water. The more efficient nature of ionized water may carry these metals and poisons deep into the cellular matrix, to act as potential time bombs later as they accumulate over time.

Water catalysts generally may make water more hydrating; however they are hardly universal in their health support function. Electrons, alkalinity, hexagonal structuring or micro clustering are all buzz words commonly in use. Truth is, most water catalysts have either no energy, negative energy or undesired stimulatory energy. You want none of these in your body. One water catalyst tested claimed increased electron activity. It had only a 3% increase. That does not justify the $40 price tag on the 8 oz bottle. On the other hand, examples like QuantaWater, Perfect Balance and Harmony Drops are some of the top water catalysts on the market. These offer affordable, very high vibrational harmonic support when small amounts are added to any pure water, plus they make the water nearly perfect in its hydration. You must make your own choices. You can also check www.ewater.com or www.energywater.com regularly to keep up on what is available. www.wellnesslecture.com has solid lectures on water, air and energies. Use lsi@wellnesslecture.com as a referring email to get into wellnesslecture.com and enjoy the wealth of knowledge contained within.

Whole home filtration is a solid choice for those who are willing to put their health as a top priority.

Water softeners should only be used in exceptionally hard water, and they should be used with chlorine and chemical removing filter. They can be very harmful to our environment, and there are excellent electronic alternatives today.

Whole home filters can contain:
- Carbon (may be catalytic, activated, or multiple purpose)
- Carbon and magnetics
- Carbon, magnetics, far infrared and harmonic technology
- Electronic Water softening
- Salt Regenerated Water Softening (When extreme hardness is present)

Each has its strengths and limitations, and should combine a reverse osmosis for the drinking and cooking water at the kitchen sink. A VitalizerPlus appliance combines very well with the reverse osmosis system. Water for the whole home does not have to be the quality needed for the internal function of our bodies. If it were that pure, it would leach copper and lead from the plumbing. For bathing and showering, washing clothes and flushing toilets, we need volatile chemicals, chlorine, and chlorine by-products removed. Fluoride is not absorbed through the skin and does not easily vaporize in a shower or bath. Salts and dead dirt minerals also are not absorbed. These all are only a hazard once inside the body on a regular basis.

Swimming Pools and Spas can be treated energetically now with great positive results for the body. Although costly equipment can reduce the use of chlorine and algaecides, there is no such thing as a maintenance free pool. Concentrate on a healthy pool, not maintenance free. Use www.ewater.com as a resource for Pools and Spas.

SILVER HYDROSOL: A NATURAL HEALTH REMEDY

IS THERE ANYTHING I CAN DO TO BETTER PREPARE OR PROTECT MY FAMILY FROM VIRUS'S, HEAVY METALS, TOXINS, PATHOGENS OR FORCED VACCINATIONS...AND WHAT IF MY CHILDREN OR I HAVE HAD VACCINATIONS IN THE PAST?

Knowing that we have some safe, natural and powerful solutions available to help safeguard us in this ever so increasingly dangerous chemical, microbial and pathogenic resistant and persistent era in which we live can sure bring us some much needed comfort and self health empowerment.

(Colloidal) Silver Hydrosol (Anti-microbial, Anti-inflammatory, Anti-fungal, Immune Support & Healing Accelerator.
(Colloidal) Silver Hydrosol, a safe, natural, immune support and illness conquering solution is addressing a wide array of health deterrents

and is a shining example of Mother Nature at her best. A high quality silver solution like Silver Hydrosol is one of the greatest defensive and preventive remedies we have available.

Hundreds of studies conducted over the past 90 years at top medical universities in both Europe and America have confirmed the phenomenal infection fighting powers of this safe, all-natural anti-microbial substance. In ancient times, the first metals discovered and used were gold, copper and silver.

Silver has reportedly been shown to be extremely beneficial against the fight of many illness causing micro-organisms, safely, quite rapidly and without causing any interactions while taking other natural or modern products. Viruses and bacteria reportedly do not become immune to or develop mutant or resistant strains when silver is used. Silver has been used with excellent results under the most demanding health care circumstances for nearly a century. It is clearly making a dramatic comeback as one of the stars of modern society, and it may just turn out to be the answer to today's horrifying crisis of infectious, resistant strains of pathogenic micro-organisms. Since its discovery, silver has been touted to have saved more lives from deadly infections than any other substance in existence!

There is a long documented history of the efficacy of silver use and a great deal of scientific studies and the following are just a few examples.

Silver has been for thousands of years highly regarded as a versatile healing tool. Silver was used in ancient Greece, Phoenicia, Macedonia and Rome, quite widely to control infections and spoiling foods. Even Hippocrates, the "Father of Medicine," taught that silver healed wounds and controlled disease. Silver nitrate was noted in the contemporary Roman pharmacopoeia in 69 B.C. The Elder, Pliny in A.D. 78 Natural History makes the statement in Book XXXIII, Section XXXV, that the slag of silver "...has healing properties as an ingredient in plasters, being extremely effective in causing wounds to close up..." Throughout the Middle East silver was used medicinally from A.D. 700 - 980 for heart conditions, blood purification processes and halitosis.

Pioneers of the American West dropped silver dollars in containers of milk and water to help keep it fresh and protect from bacteria and algae. During the wars with Napoleon, the armies of Tsar Alexander used water casks lined with silver to clean drinking water from rivers and streams. The Imperial Russian army was also known for doing this during World War I and some units of the Soviet Army during World War II. Today all branches of the military use silver lined water backpacks.

What is believed to be the first clinical description of water-purifying or the cleansing effect by silver was noted and recorded by Raulin in 1869. Raulin also observed that Aspergillus Niger could not grow in silver vessels.

Searle, A.B. The use of Colloids in Health and Disease. The British Medical Journal. November, 1913, p. 83 Dr. Henry Crookes. Colloidal Silver is proven particularly effective in cases of intestinal troubles. Dr. Henry Crooks found that Silver in the colloidal state is highly germicidal, quite harmless to humans and absolutely nontoxic. Rather than in a chemical compound, the Silver, in the colloidal state, may be applied in a much more concentrated form, with correspondingly better results.

All fungus, virus, bacterium, streptococcus, staphylococcus, and other pathogenic organisms are killed in three or four minutes; in fact, there is no microbe tested that was not killed by Colloidal Silver in six minutes or less, using a dilution of as little as five parts per million, though there are no side effects whatsoever from high concentrations. "Use of Colloids in Health and Disease," quoted in "Report: Colloidal Silver," Health Consciousness, Vol. 15, No.4.

Quoting, Dr. Richard Davies, The Silver Institute, Wash, Vol. 18, 4, p. 295. "Silver, Our Mightiest Germ Fighter," Science Digest, March 1978. As an antibiotic, colloidal silver kills over 650 disease causing organisms, and resistant strains fail to develop. Silver is the best all-around germ fighter we have and is absolutely non-toxic! Doctors report that, taken internally, it works against syphilis, cholera, malaria, diabetes and severe burns. Bio Tech News 1995 Richard L. Davies, executive director of the Silver Institute which monitors silver technology in 37 countries, reports: "In four years we've described 87 important new medical uses for silver."

"Colloidal Preparations of Silver in Pharmacy," British Medical Journal, February 1923: "Pure Silver is entirely non-irritant. In tests at very high concentrations, it has been shown repeatedly that the rapidly exerted disinfectant action is of considerable therapeutic value."

Colloidal Silver has long been recognized by medical experts as one of the most potent antidotes on earth for food poisoning. Colloidal Silver easily killed e-coli food poisoning bacterium reported in 1928 by a researcher named Schweizer. In 1937 a researcher named Mallman confirmed that silver ions killed e-coli. In 1982, Dr. J. Cowlishaw again confirmed the effectiveness of electrically generated colloidal silver against e-coli and other microorganisms associated with food poisoning. Dr. Bjorn Nordstrom, of the Karolinska Institute, Sweden, has used silver in his cancer treatment method. He says the whole thing is quite simple. This brought rapid remission in patients given up on by other doctors.

Colloidal silver was one of the few substances on earth that was successfully used against anthrax and other plague like pathogens in the early 1900's prior to the advent of modern day antibiotics as verified by the book, Colloids In Biology And Medicine, by H. Beckhold, pages 364 thru 376. According to researcher James South, MA., as early as 1887 a number of researchers had discovered that silver both in the liquid solution and as an airborne aerosol was toxic to deadly anthrax spores. (Ref: N. Grier, Silver and Its Compounds in Disinfection, Sterilization and Preservation, S. Block ed., Philadelphia: Lea& Febiger, 1983, pp. 380-428; H. Beckhold, Colloids in Biology and Medicine, N.Y.,: D. Van Nostrand, 1919, pp. 364-376; Anti-Aging Bulletin, International Anti-Aging Systems, Vol. 4, Issue 3, April-May, 1999, "Hi Yo Silver Away!" by James South, M.A.)

Dr. Robert Becker is probably one of the most well known Colloidal Silver researchers and is also a bestselling author. Dr. Robert O. Becker,

Orthopedic Surgeon, and Noted Biomedical Researcher From Syracuse Medical University and bestselling author wrote, "Silver did more than kill disease causing organisms, it promoted major growth of bone, and accelerated the healing of injured tissues by over 50%! He also found that silver stimulates healing in the skin and other soft tissues in a way unlike any known natural process. Silver deficiency was responsible for the improper functioning of the immune system. Burn patients and even elderly patients notice more rapid healing. Dr. Becker also discovered that all cancer cells change back to normal cells and virtually all strains of pathogens resistant to pharmaceutical antibiotics are killed by silver! He also discovered that the silver was promoting a new kind of cell growth which looked like the cells of children!" These cells grew fast, he wrote "producing a diverse and surprising assortment of primitive cell forms able to multiply at a great rate then differentiate into the specific cells of an organ or tissue that had been injured, even in patients over 50 years old. "In no case were undesirable side-effects of the silver treatment apparent. Dr. Becker also discovered that a silver impregnated nylon dressing attached to a small battery would cause previously untreatable osteomyelitis and bones that refuse to knit to heal quickly. This combination of silver and tiny electric currents worked so well that it is a standard practice today, when broken bones refuse to knit, to use Dr. Becker's electrified silver process.

References: Treatment of Orthopedic Infections with Electrically Generated Silver Ions. The Journal of Bone and Joint Surgery, American Volume, October, 1978. Vol. 60-A, No.7. Dr. Robert Becker, "The Body Electric and Cross Currents," recognized a correlation between low silver levels and sickness. He said the silver deficiency was responsible for the improper functioning of the immune system. Becker, R. & Selden, G. (1985). The Body Electric: Electromagnetism and the Foundation of Life. New York, NY:

Today silver is used commonly by many of the major airlines to prevent bacterial contamination to the water supply. The U.S. (NASA) and Russian space shuttle vehicles both use silver and copper water filtration and purification systems. Silver is also used in thousands of spas and swimming pools around the country to kill the growth of harmful microbes. Subway and train stations in London and other parts of the UK are considering using a powerful, non-toxic colloidal silver disinfectant spray to help fend off the spread of the flu virus this winter after Hong Kong subways recently announced its use of the spray.

The MTR Company revealed its plan to use nano silver-titanium dioxide coating (NSTDC) spray on most surfaces on the Hong Kong metro rail system. Roughly 2.5 million commuters ride the Hong Kong rail system every day, and can easily spread colds and the flu through common surfaces. The NSTDC disinfectant spray has been certified as effective at killing wide ranges of bacteria, mold and viruses, including the H1N1 virus. MTR announced it would be sprayed on all escalator handrails, Add Value machines, the buttons on ticket issuing machines and all handrails and buttons in elevators in the company's Hong Kong stations. The colloidal silver spray would also be applied to all grab poles and straps within the trains. I don't know about you but this article tells me to be sure to bring along your Colloidal Silver whenever you travel.

Silver is well established in the Japanese market place, which places a high importance on antimicrobial protection. Silver ions are supported in an inorganic matrix or substrate such as zeolites or alumina-silica-based biocides used to protect consumers, especially in hospital settings where containment of disease transmission is of much concern. The Japanese are forward thinking in terms of technology and demand for protection and the method in which silver particles are delivered.

There is nothing like this on the planet. No other supplement, mineral, herb or food has the instant, fast acting power and endless capabilities and vast uses that premium Colloidal Silver solutions like Silver Hydrosol have, nor has any other - touted to have saved as many lives. Once you experience it you'll never want to go without it (unprotected) again.

There have been many reports of people spraying Silver solutions in children's eyes for Pink Eye or any eye infections, vision problems, accidents and for preventative measures successfully. Doctors have been putting a form of silver called silver nitrate in baby's eyes immediately after birth for many, many years to safely kill bacteria and any virus that may have been subjected to the eyes in the birth canal. This has worked wonderfully well and many doctors still do this today. As a matter of fact, if we used the more advanced forms of Colloidal Silver now available I believe we would see even greater results in protecting not only the vision but all areas health.

*Using Silver Hydrosol now, BEFORE YOU GET ILL OR VACCINATED, is vital for preparing, strengthening and boosting the immune system and providing a certain level of protection against flus, pathogens and dangerous microbes. Remember it only stays in your system for a short time so I would take small amounts often and more if I did happen to come down with something. **STOCK UP NOW**, because it will not be readily available during an emergency due to extreme demand and by the time you finally get it, it will be too late!

Is Zeolite Really A Cancer Cure? Does it kill viruses and is it safe to use for chelation (detoxing & cleansing) Heavy Metals and Toxins?
Zeolites have been used as health supplements for thousands of years and can even remove radioactive contaminants. Uranium is of grave concern and the use of Uranium weapons has caused a global diabetes epidemic since 1991 according to scientist Leuren Moret. It is enough uranium dust to cause an estimated twenty five million additional cancers in Iraq in the next decade. The US and UK military still use uranium munitions. There are only 24 million Iraqis and many now have multiple cancers.

It is estimated that 1 in 3 women and 1 in 2 men will get cancer before they are 75.

Although it certainly seems as if Zeolite cures Cancer and many other so called diseases, but really it is your own body and the immune system that does this. Here is how it works. Clinoptilolite Zeolite in its cage like structure attracts, encapsulates and effectively eliminates the body burden of toxic heavy metals, neurotoxins and free radicals. Not only does it de-chemicalize, but the Clinoptilolite Zeolite with the added

Humic and Fulvic Acids (now being called miracle minerals) actually re-mineralizes and nourishes the cells and is not only being used during sickness, but also as a powerful preventative and immune and health boosting solution. This is the most advanced form of Zeolite there is today. Liquid Zeolite with Humic/Fulvic Acids and a new powerful Molecular Silver functions as a natural chelator drawing in through its magnetic field toxic metals like Cadmium, Mercury, Lead, Arsenic, etc. and storing them in its cage like structure and then begins with handling the pesticides and on through to the potentially pathogenics and pathogenic virus and bacteria neutralizing and safely carrying them out of the body with no stress on the liver or other organs and also as a powerful anti-viral. This is a very unique formula and it is only available from one source that I know of.

The Zeolite Humic/Fulvic Molecular Silver Formula can safely be used on babies, adults, animals and every single one of the aforementioned should be on this formula if we expect to survive and bear healthy babies. With this formula you are being re-mineralized with RARE "FINITE" ancient and prehistoric trace plant minerals. This formula can be safely taken alongside any other regimen you may be doing. There are no known interactions.

Other chelators like plain Zeolites acting alone, EDTA, foot baths and patches can remove vital minerals, relocate or scatter toxins and the result can be quite dangerous if not monitored closely. Reports of people becoming terribly ill after a few foot bath sessions, I believe, is partly do to the poisons and toxins that are not removed at the time, being scattered about, relocated and then left for the already taxed liver and elimination system to deal with. Zeolite actually encapsulates toxins and heavy metals making them harmless, even while still in the body. So, as the body eliminates these encapsulated poisons there is no stress or strain on the organs and thus no detox ramifications. If you are using any of the other above techniques I would definitely add this Zeolite formula to the regimen because it will also provide you with the much needed trace minerals directly to the cells via the Fulvic Acid molecule.

1. **Fulvic Acid Is One Of Nature's Most Powerful Life Restorers.** The Fulvic Acid Group, natural organic electrolytes, can balance, activate and energize the biological properties with whatever organic material it comes into contact. An electrolyte is soluble in water or any other similar medium able to conduct electrical current. The power of an electrolyte has been shown to have the ability to restore life in repeated tests on animal cells (giant amoebae) in what astonished researchers termed "a beautiful demonstration." When the electrolyte potential was removed during the test, the cell ruptured, disintegrated into the surrounding fluid and died. When electrical potential was reintroduced, the cell reconstructed and returned to healthy activity!

2. **Fulvic Acid Promotes Electro-Chemical Balance Whether Donor Or Receptor.** Electro-chemical balance is required for health in any organic system or body. Fulvic Acid is available at times as an electron donor and at other times as an electron acceptor, based on the cell's requirements for balance.

3. **Fulvic Acid Dissolves Minerals & Trace Elements.** Fulvic Acid actively dissolves minerals and metals when in solution with water. Metallic minerals simply dissolve into the fulvic structure and become bio-chemically reactive and-mobile.

4. **Fulvic Acid Forms Complex Molecular Structures.** The Fulvic Acid actually transforms these minerals and metals into elaborate Fulvic Acid complex molecular structures that have vastly different characteristics from their previous metallic mineral form.

5. **Fulvic Acid Enhances Availability.** Fulvic Acid enhances the availability of nutrients and makes them more readily absorbable. It also allows minerals to regenerate and prolongs the residence time of essential nutrients.

6. **Fulvic Acid Catalyzes Enzyme Reactions** Fulvic Acid can also increase enzyme activity and act as both a donor or as an acceptor to supply electro-chemical balance to a cell. It increases the activity of several enzymes such as transaminase, invertase and alkaline phosphates.

7. **Fulvic Acid Increases Assimilation.** Fulvic Acid metal organic complexes are relatively heavy and because of this, they have small molecular size and can easily penetrate cells.

8. **Fulvic Acid Stimulates Metabolism.** Fulvic Acid appears to cause the genetic mechanism of plants to function at a higher level. Any means by which plant cells are exposed to Fulvic Acid can improve growth. Oxygen is absorbed more intensely in the presence of Fulvic Acids.

9. **Fulvic Acid Detoxifies Pollutants** An important quality of humic substances is related to their sorptive interaction with environmental chemicals either before or after they reach concentrations toxic to living organisms. The toxic herbicide known as Paraquat is rapidly detoxified by humic substances (Fulvic Acid).

10. **Fulvic Acid Increases Metabolism Of Proteins.** Fulvic Acid intensifies the metabolism of proteins, RNA and DNA. Fulvic Acid definitely increases DNA content in cells and increases and enhances the rate of RNA synthesis.

Humic Acid Research

It is only recently that scientific research has been performed on humic acid. It is a large, long-chain molecule that can be isolated in a relatively pure form from the soil's humate layer. Scientific studies have shown that it impairs the attachment of the HIV-1 virus, one of the viruses responsible for the development of AIDS. Herpes simplex virus infections have been found to be impeded. Another study examined influenza viruses, including the swine flu, with the same results. Exotic viruses like the West Nile Virus, Hemorrhagic Fever and Coxsackie viruses have been found to be inhibited by humic acid. There is every reason to expect that its antiviral properties are broad spectrum, meaning it may have usefulness against the Asian or bird flu pandemic. The mechanism of action of humic acid in these cases is believed to be the blockage of a virus particle from attaching to and entering a healthy cell. Viruses can't replicate or divide without entering and taking over the cell's DNA for the making of more virus particles. By keeping one virus particle from becoming thousands, it effectively blocks the infection from happening.

Humic acid has also been scientifically shown to be a free radical scavenger.

Free radicals are "broken" molecules that are off-balanced from the standpoint of having too many electrons on them. They are dangerous to healthy, living cells. Free radicals can interfere with our DNA and the effect can be cancer causing. By binding them up, humic acid makes free radicals safe from us. Humic acid is a potent chelator as well. A chelator is a molecule that binds metals, including toxic heavy metals. It is able to scavenge for these heavy metals and eliminate them from the body. It seems to increase the permeability of cell walls, allowing for easier transfer of nutrient metals. Research indicates that humic acid can bind to essential metals as well; much like soil humic acid did millions of years ago it can provide nutrients to living things growing in the soil. It's felt that by binding to healthy metals, humic acid can aid in their absorption in the body.

Humic acid also seems to modulate or regulate the effects of our stress hormones.

Because of its size, it likely blocks the stress hormones from reaching the receptor site. Interestingly, a study out of Penn State found that rats with humic acid showed much lower levels of stress hormones than those that didn't. Our immune system, too, reaps the benefits of humic acid.

Humates can increase polysaccharide sugars in our body which bind to Killer T Cells (immune killer cells) and facilitate communication between the Killer T Cells and other body cells.

The function of Killer T cells is then modulated by the polysaccharides. Excessive Killer T Cell function in the body is part of what facilitates auto-immune diseases like rheumatoid arthritis. Humic acid has anti-inflammatory properties. While its full effect is not understood, it has been shown to diminish cervical inflammation in subjects with cervicitis. In the years before we depleted our growing soil, humic acid was a natural part of the food chain. Without it, we're missing something that seems to have healthful benefits against viruses, heavy metal toxicity and dangerous free radicals.

When you remove the toxins and poisons the body accumulates on a daily basis the body can then naturally and much more effectively heal and regenerate. Quite simply put—remove the garbage and the flies leave! *We live on a chemically polluted planet and it and all of its inhabitants desperately need urgent help and intervention if we are going to survive. We can heal, save this planet and ourselves if we wake up now.* We find ourselves now living in an era where each and every one of us is toxic and bombarded with heavy metals and chemicals. We find ourselves having to detoxify on an ongoing daily basis to remove the onslaught of toxins we breathe in with every breath (75,000 micro clustered chemicals), shower in and eat. I don't care who you are or where you are on this planet you are going to be taking in chemicals every day...period.

These dangerous chemicals and heavy metals prevent you from being able to properly utilize nutrients, vitamins, and minerals, and so, you become severely deficient, diseased, degenerated (loss of energy) and rapidly age—thus dying needlessly. You go to the store and buy hundreds of dollars worth of herbs, supplements and minerals looking for something to help and nothing does. WHY? Because, you must remove the toxins and poisons FIRST. You have accumulated a wide array of toxins and heavy metals and if you have them in your mouth (amalgam fillings) or anywhere else in your environment that is within your control remove them. Please do not expect to completely detoxify in a few days or weeks with a couple of bottles of Zeolite. This is a safe, slow detox the way it should be, so be persistent and do this now. Do not wait or stockpile this without using it as well. A healthy, detoxified and strong immune system will be your best defense for flus, vaccinations and all health threats. If you or anyone you know gets the vaccinations, or has had them in the past, detoxify with liquid Zeolite Plus (humic/fulvic silver) and drink ionic silver hydrosol often. Also take plenty of chlorella, blue green algae, Vitamin C, lots of Vitamin D (best source is our sun) before and after the shots. Obviously, a good organic diet with plenty of nutrient dense fruits and vegetables is a given. Drink ½ your body weight in ounces of PURE water daily and get 7 – 8 hours of sleep which will aid in the healing, repair and regeneration processes that occur during deep sleep.

The following is an excerpt from a study made public by the National Institutes of Health (NIH) on The Broad-Spectrum Antiviral Efficacy of Natural and Synthetic Humates (Humic/Fulvic Acids). This Report presents the results of toxicology, cell proliferation, and efficacy testing work carried out on natural-product and synthetic humate materials in 2001-2002 by contract laboratories of the Virology Branch of the Antiviral Research and Antimicrobial Chemistry Program (Dr. Christopher Tseng, Program Officer), Division of Microbiology and Infectious Diseases (DMID) Screening and Testing Program for Antiviral, Immunomodulatory, Antitumor and/or Drug Delivery Activities, National Institutes of Allergy and Infectious Diseases (NIAID), under the auspices of the National Institutes of Health (NIH, Bethesda, Maryland).

Efficacy data are presented for five herpes viruses, three influenza viruses, and two hemorrhagic fever viruses. Results…

The efficacy data for all humates with the five herpes viruses examined in this work are provided in the following tables. Not all are shown here. As shown, synthetic humates CA and HGA were found to be effective against HSV-1 and HSV-2, and their efficacy approached that of Acyclovir. Humate CA was somewhat effective against human cytomegalovirus, while synthetic HGA was equally so against Varicella Zoster virus. Humate CA was very highly effective against Epstein-Barr virus.

The efficacy data for all humates with the influenza viruses examined in this work are provided in the following tables. Not all are shown here. As shown, synthetic humate CA and natural-product humate HA were found to be quite effective against all three influenza viruses. In addition, the potency of synthetic CA exceeded that of Ribavirin in two of the three strains tested. In the time of addition studies (Table XVII), the most efficacious antiviral effect was observed when cells were pre-treated (at time 0) with humates, that is, the humates appeared to prevent infection. In addition, activity was also present with post-infection treatment regimens (Ribavirin lost all its antiviral activity by 24 h). For example, at 100 μg/mL concentration of humates CA and HA in infected cells, discrete virus foci were seen that appeared like small plaques (particularly when the drugs were added 24 hours after virus exposure).

These results suggest that the compounds also inhibited virus adsorption even after the infection process had begun. (Mature influenza virus buds out of the host cell, then goes on to infect new cells during its life cycle. Since the cells were continuously exposed to the humate materials, newly-formed virus exiting cells during the early rounds of virus replication would be blocked from attaching and entering uninfected cells to initiate new infections.)

Although only one humate material was employed against a single influenza strain in this work, the data nevertheless indicate that humates do in fact show some promise as potential influenza inhibitors.

The efficacy data for all humate materials with the hemorrhagic fever viruses examined in this work are provided in the following tables. As shown, the humates exhibited substantial efficacy against both hemorrhagic fever viruses, synthetic CA and natural-product HA particularly so against Punta Toro A virus. The addition of humates 1 hour before virus exposure, at the time of virus exposure, and 1 hour after virus exposure resulted in similar levels of inhibition of viral infection.

The US Food and Drug Association (FDA) have given zeolite a G.R.A.S. rating which means Generally Recognized As Safe. Zeolite powder is approved and widely used as a supplement for livestock to improve animal health and production.

World's First Home Use Heavy Metal Test.

An inexpensive Heavy Metal Home Use Test is now available that will tell you your level of toxicity in a few minutes! This is a very valuable test that gives us more control over our most precious health. You are toxic! Test your children. This test also works great to track your detox progress so you know when to drop down to a maintenance dose. If this test shows you have a high level of heavy metals then your health is rapidly failing. This measures the free metal ions in the urine and is quite accurate. This level of toxicity measured directly relates to your current level of health. This test should be done often and you can also use it to test your drinking water to see if your filtration system is working properly at removing heavy metals and chemicals. Eliminating intake of these in our water is within our control and is vital.

Widespread Vitamin D and Mineral Deficiencies are alarming and even more so in our children. The few minerals they are getting they are unable to absorb due to the cell receptor sites being plugged with Heavy Metals like Mercury, Cadmium, Arsenic, Aluminum and various chemicals, pesticides and even fuels. We are literally minerally starved. Recent studies are even finding rocket fuel in 100% of breast milk samples taken from women across 18 states.

There are planes flying overhead dropping payloads of chemicals on the food crops to kill bugs at this very moment. Every insect in its path is destroyed as we hover inside with our pets and loved ones keeping all doors and windows tightly closed. This is absolute madness, when will it end? When will we be enlightened and advance to a higher level of consciousness? Each and every one of us must take responsibility and do our part. If half of us that are currently accepting chemicals stopped purchasing and using these chemicals, refused to eat chemical laced food and returned all chemicals in our possession for a refund or at least for proper disposal the chemical companies would go broke! One big problem solved.

As long as we continue to buy the poison and poisonous products, they will remain. Big Agri-business is not going to suddenly develop a consciousness and stop manufacturing and spewing chemicals into and onto everything. The same is true for the heavy metals, viruses and poisons in the vaccinations, and I simply say...NO THANK YOU.

We take in 75,000 micro clustered chemicals with every single breath we take! Folks you also need Enzymes not only as a result of this but most of us don't eat a raw nutrient dense diet. Our gastrointestinal systems are failing—we are not digesting our food. Helping America has a very unique, high quality, fermented liquid enzyme product shipped with extreme care and caution from Korea. This is unlike anything you will find anywhere else. It is made from 100 wild plants from deep recesses high in the mountains and then the entire plant with seed and fruit is naturally fermented for over a year in large vats. The end result is a rich and nutritious liquid high in natural vitamins, minerals and enzymes. This is a vital and absolute necessity for regenerating our polluted, deficient bodies while providing all of the enzymes we need in the right form for proper utilization. This is top shelf folks.

We can change our destiny.

We must educate ourselves and learn to be self sufficient, help others and raise our level of consciousness and spirituality. We are not helpless. We are very powerful, more powerful than you know and it all comes from within, do not look outside. If we are not healthy, this is almost impossible to do. It is absolutely critical you maintain optimum health and show others how to do the same. If our brain is full of Mercury then we are weak and unable to focus, living a meager existence, helping no one and burdening many. It's time we wake up and get out of the fog.

The Silver Hydrosol, Zeolite Plus Cellular Silver, Liquid Enzymes and Humic/Fulvic Minerals from Helping America are rich premium grade advanced forms which feeds our cells thus allowing our immune systems to heal, strengthen and protect us. Their Zeolite is 100% organically formulated and cleaned Zeolite. Many others are claiming to be, but don't fall for it. Helping America's formulator has 30 years in the business and is the only one that has developed this natural cleaning process and it is a highly guarded trade secret! If it's cheap it's fake and many are using chemicals and questionable practices. The combination of these 4 items taken together and consistently is a power house that will lift you to new heights. You will feel and see the results! The Heavy Metal Test then backs up the detox part and confirms that it's working and keeps you abreast of the progress!! Please test your children for Heavy Metals and their level of toxicity. Detoxify and cleanse accordingly so that their immune systems can once again function correctly for proper development. I hope I have established the grave importance of these things and that you understand why we need them.

*The forward thinking Sun+Rite Company located on the island of Maui have chosen Helping America's Silver Hydrosol to be the main ingredient in their entire line of natural skin care and antiseptics. Their preliminary testing, feedback and experience formulating and incorporating the premium Hydrosol with high quality organic essential oils has shown phenomenal results.

I personally use Helping America's Silver Hydrosol and have for quite some time now. My family, friends and all those I love and care about are using this Silver and seeing wonderful results. I carry some of this with me and when I was practicing I recommended it to my patients, and so do my student MD's like Dr. Hohn or Dr. Crone, which by the way we have seen it easily beat Lyme Disease. The well known medical scientist Dr. Paul Farber contracted Lyme Disease in the early 90's and also cured himself of Lyme Disease quickly with Colloidal Silver. Another example of amazing healing power applies to burns of all types. Simply spray on a burn and immediately experience pain lessoning and some people have even said they can see new skin forming and have witnessed rapid healing with no scarring, infection or pain whatsoever!

Children love this feature.

It is my belief, that if our emergency response personnel were armed with Silver Hydrosol and used it properly we would see huge drops in infection rates, rapidly increased healing and much less suffering from pain. This is something we need to work on.

This is the only Silver and Zeolite product that I promote and endorse. I do so freely with absolutely no payment or personal benefit what so ever. I do not sell or accept any payments for my recommendations. Kevin, the owner and founder of Helping America is always there to assist and answer my friends' and my questions. This is quite rare now because with most companies, you must talk to a machine or an ordering department. Kevin has over 10 years experience with this Silver Hydrosol, as well as some other wonderful health benefiting products. I know Kevin, his family and his pets all personally use these products.

It's comforting to know that we have safe, natural and powerful solutions to help safeguard us in this ever so increasingly dangerous chemical, microbial and pathogenic resistant and persistent era in which we live.

Whatever the mind of man can conceive and bring itself to believe—it can achieve. (Napoleon Hill)

What ever frequency your brain puts out, it will attract back and it will defy all physical laws. The Law of Attraction is a senior law that trumps all others. (Kevin Trudeau)

Through proper education we can learn how to protect and grow ourselves, our loved ones, our pets, our water and even our foods. Maintaining an open, clear, cleansed and healthy inquiring mind is crucial.

Contact Helping America

www.helpingamericanow.com

Toll free 877-743-5746

If you have unlimited long

Distance please use local number

507-847-4139

Bibliography

1. Seffner, W. "Effects of humic acid on the availability of iodine in the food, investigated with the histometric assessment of the thyroid gland." Conference Paper Mengen- und spurenelemente-15 Arbelstagund, 1995.

2. Bernacci, F. et al. "In vivo and in vitro mutagenicity studies on natural humic acid." Conference paper 37, Riunione scientifica, October 1991.

3. Gau, R. et al. "Induction of oxidative stress by humic acid through increasing intracellular iron; a possible mechanism leading to atherothrombotic vascular disorder in blackfoot disease." Biochem Biophys Res Commun, 2001; Vol 283; Issue 4: 743-49.

4. Iubitskaia , NS . "Sodium humate in the treatment of osteoarthritis patients." Vopr Kurortol Fizioter Lech Fiz Kult, 1999; Issue 5, 22-24.

5. Schiller, F. "Results of an oriented clinical trial of ammonium humate for the local treatment of herpesvirus hominis (HVH) infections." Dermatol Monatsschr, 1979, Vol. 165; Issue 7; 505-09.

6. Riede, U.N. "Humate induced activation of human granulocytes. Virchows Arch B Cell Pathol Incl Mol Pathol, 1991; Issue 1: 27-34.

7. Herzig, I. "The effect of sodium humate on cadmium deposition in the organs of chickens." Vet Med, 1994, Vol 39; Issue 4; 175-85.

8. Hampi, I, et al. "Pharmacokinetics of sodium humate in chickens." Vet Med, 1994; Vol 39, Issue 6; 305-313.

9. Schneider, J, et al. "Inhibition of HIV-1 in cell culture by synthetic humate analogues derived from hydroquinone; mechanism of inhibition." Virology, 1996; Vol 218, Issue 2, 389-95.

10. Thiel, KD, et al. "In vitro studies of the antiviral activity of ammonium humate against herpes simplex virus type 1 and type 2." Zentralbl Bakteriol, 1977; Vol. 239, Issue 3, 304-321.

11. Laub, R. "The chemically induced inhibition of HSV infection." Laub BioChem Corp., August 1998.

12. Laub, R. "The chemically induced inhibition of HIV-1 replication." Laub BioChem Corp., January 1995.

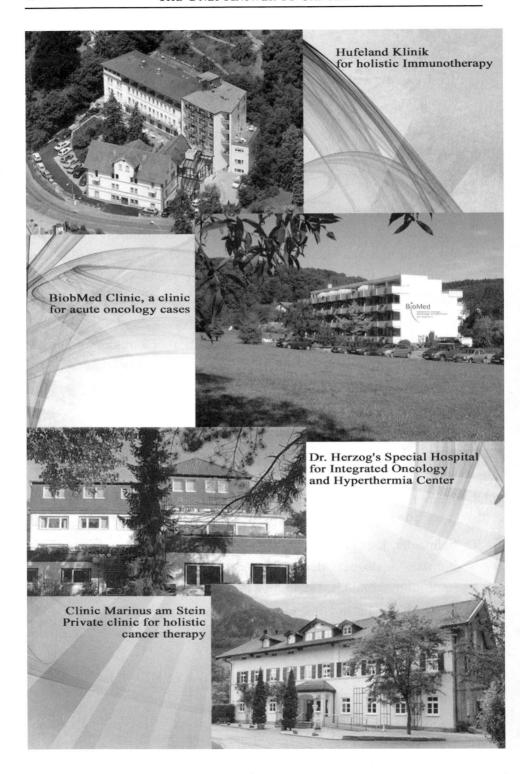

Hufeland Klinik for holistic Immunotherapy

BiobMed Clinic, a clinic for acute oncology cases

Dr. Herzog's Special Hospital for Integrated Oncology and Hyperthermia Center

Clinic Marinus am Stein Private clinic for holistic cancer therapy

THE WORLD'S BEST CANCER TREATMENTS IN EUROPE

For those who cannot or do or not want to do it all on their own here are some Cancer treatment clinics. Since most of the really effective and natural cancer cures and treatments that have no negative effects and are all natural, are forbidden in America, you have to go to Germany. Soon IBMS™ practitioners and therapists will be available for you too. Also you can order the IBMS™ home study course: IBMS-Healing Life™

The late best-selling author, physician, and medical maverick Dr. Robert Atkins, M.D., once said: "There is not one, but many cures for cancer available. But they are all being systematically suppressed by the American Cancer Society, the National Cancer Institute, and the major oncology centers. They have too much of an interest in the status quo."

Well, there you have it. Cures for cancer are available, but you don't know about them because too much money is at stake for those who want you to submit to the old-fashioned, harsh, and obsolete cancer treatment methods. It's a shame that effective cancer cures are so hard to find in America. But there's no conspiracy to suppress these cancer cures in Germany. German doctors routinely use these cures to help "terminal" cancer patients get rid of their cancer—including American patients who fly to Germany for treatment.

We Americans pride ourselves on being Number One. After all, we're the last remaining world superpower. We have the world's richest economy. We win the most gold medals at the Olympics. We have the world's best space program—the only one that has actually put men on the moon, not just once but six times. And we have the world-famous Mayo Clinic and other top-notch medical centers. Many would say we have the best health care *in the world*.

Why, then, are so many Americans from all walks of life—from movie stars to people who can't afford health insurance—going to Germany for cancer treatment and for other medical care? Since as you probably know I am originally from Germany before I became a proud American citizen, I know all these different forms of cancer treatments first hand. But first here are some names of some celebrities who've benefited from German therapies:

- Ronald Reagan
- Liz Taylor
- Cher
- Suzanne Somers
- Roy of "Siegfried and Roy"
- Jack Cassidy (the bass player from the Jefferson Airplane rock group)
- George Hamilton
- Red Buttons and his wife Alicia

Hopeless Patient Lives 29 Years

Alicia Buttons was diagnosed with cancer in 1972. Her American doctors gave her terrible news; she had an advanced case of one of the most dreaded cancers: oral pharyngeal cancer. Surgery for this kind of cancer can leave the patient with a disfigured face. The doctors told Alicia Buttons that her cancer was hopeless and terminal. They said, "With luck, you might be able to live a year." But Red and his wife didn't take that American doctor's death sentence as the gospel truth. Instead, Red took his wife to Germany for mild, gentle alternative treatments that are non-toxic. And she lived for 29 more years.

From Near Death To Driving A Mercedes

I'm sure you heard about what happened to Roy Horn of "Siegfried and Roy" on October 3, 2003. Apparently Roy stumbled or had some kind of seizure on stage and his white tiger picked Roy up by the neck as a mother cat picks up her kittens. This bite caused severe damage. Many people believed Roy's career was over. He was making hardly any improvement in American hospitals. So in June, 2005, he went to a clinic in Germany for alternative treatments. By May, 2007, Roy was testing out his new Mercedes at Little Bavaria. He announced to the public, "Look at me now—I am back, better than ever." Following the devastating tiger attack, who would have ever thought that Roy would be back "better than ever"—in his own words?

Suzanne Somers received a little-known therapy in Germany

In 2001, actress Suzanne Somers got breast cancer at age 54. She had surgery and radiation. Her American doctors strongly recommended that she follow up these treatments with chemo. They were aghast when Suzanne said no to their chemo and instead used mistletoe injections—a German therapy. The German therapy was successful. All the top cancer doctors in Germany use mistletoe therapy to boost their patients' immune systems.

J. Lo sends her aunt with cancer to Germany

When Jennifer Lopez's aunt was losing her battle against ovarian cancer in a New York hospital, J. Lo paid for her treatment at one of Germany's finest cancer clinics. The treatments the aunt received in Germany were mild and healing. They weren't grueling and harsh like the American-style treatments that cause side effects such as baldness, nausea and violent retching, and loss of skin color.

Cher regularly goes to a German clinic for health tune-ups.

The Hypocrisy of the American Cancer Establishment

Executives at organizations such as the American Cancer Society and agencies such as the U.S. Food and Drug Administration (FDA) strongly recommend that *a patient* undergoes the traditional American treatment. These treatments have never shown any significant cures. In fact, the cut, poison and burn usually kills the patient if it does not cure him, it also destroys the patient's quality of life and life expectancy, in my observations.

What happens when one of them gets cancer? You'd think they'd practice what they preach when *they* get cancer, right? Wrong!

Back in 1987 a man named Jeff Harsh, who was working on a video documentary, interviewed one of Germany's top cancer physicians, Dr. Hans Nieper, M.D. (1928-1998). Dr. Nieper helped his patients get rid of cancer by using alternative methods the FDA forbids in America. One of Dr. Nieper's forbidden methods was the natural substance called Laetrile, which is derived from apricot seeds.

In the interview, Dr. Nieper said, "President Reagan is a very nice man," having treated him for cancer in July of 1983. Dr. Neiper added, "You wouldn't believe how many FDA officials or relatives or acquaintances of FDA officials come to see me as patients in Hanover. You wouldn't believe this—or directors of the American Medical Association (AMA), or American Cancer Society (ACS), or the presidents of orthodox cancer institute's. That's the fact."

Well, there you have it. The wealthy executives who run the ACS, the FDA, and the AMA beat the drum for American-style cancer treatments that they recommend for you and your loved ones. But when they get cancer, well, that's different: many of them head for Germany.

But it's not just the rich and famous who go to Germany for medical treatment. You'll be shocked at how affordable the German clinics are compared to the sky-high prices American hospitals charge. Even some Americans who can't afford medical insurance find they can afford *German* medical treatment.

Why do Americans from all walks of life go to Germany for medical treatment? Well, there are at least three reasons:

American doctors say, "Nothing more can be done"—but German doctors offer a ray of hope. This is probably the most common reason so many American cancer patients choose Germany is because their American doctors have told them, "There is no hope."

Doctors in Germany know over 300 other therapies that can be done physically to rid the patient of cancer. The most effective therapists today include the Dr. Coldwell IBMS™ into their physical treatments like Dr. Thomas Hohn and Dr. Holger Crone for example, and the good news is that these German therapies are effective and non-toxic. What's more, they're amazingly inexpensive by comparison to American treatments.

I come from a strong line of healers who have been curing patients with natural methods for over 2000 years. In stark contrast to the repressive situation in the USA, all of the advanced natural therapies have the approval of Germany's health ministry, and the German government has licensed all natural and orthodox medical clinics.

Germany is the only country in the world that has in their constitution that the government has to license Natural Healers. They are NMDs, similar to medical doctors, but with training in natural healing. Both the government healthcare system and private insurance companies pay for treatment at these clinics.

Unfortunately, the typical American doctor only learns one approach to cancer treatment in medical school: the "cut-burn-poison" approach and by law has to apply it to his cancer patients. In the US, if an MD tried to cure their cancer patients with natural cures they would lose their license and would be probably thrown into jail like the doctor in California who cured his patients with B17. He went public with his success and got his license revoked and he was thrown into jail.

Most American doctors just don't know about alternative therapies. They apply what they have been brainwashed to do in medical school.

Let's stroke my heritage ego for a moment

Tragically, in America cancer treatment today isn't much different than the homicidal treatments of 60 years ago. Fortunately, the word is starting to reach many Americans that German doctors have achieved a real breakthrough in cancer treatment and in Germany it is legal to cure with natural methods, where it is against the law in America. That alone should be enough to impeach a lot of politicians for treason, at least in my opinion.

To make natural cancer cures not available in the US and even against the law is, in my opinion, waging war against the American public. Everybody that is involved in this conspiracy should be in jail. Should anyone be surprised that the Germans are arguably the finest cancer doctors in the world? Let's face it: The Germans are noted for spectacular achievements. It was German rocket scientists in Russia who launched Sputnik, which inaugurated the space age. It was German rocket scientists in America who were essential to putting men on the moon. Germans have made countless scientific and technical breakthroughs.

Here are just a few:

- In 1714 Daniel Gabriel Fahrenheit invented the mercury thermometer.

- In 1885 Karl Benz (of Mercedes-Benz fame) built the first practical car run by internal combustion, and Gottlieb Daimler invented his landmark gasoline engine.

- Rudolf Diesel invented the engine named for him

- In 1899 Felix Hoffman was the first to synthesize a medically useful form of aspirin. Bayer, a German company, manufactured Hoffman's new product.

- In 1916 Albert Einstein announced his general theory of relativity. Today the Germans make some of the world's finest cars and the finest optical products. In fact, Germany is still a top exporter of high-quality manufactured products while the United States, sadly, has slipped behind. Is it any wonder that in cancer treatment, German doctors leave most American cancer doctors in the dust?

It costs $350,000 to die of cancer in America!

Surprisingly, the second reason Americans go to Germany for cancer treatment is because some people can't afford the American cancer treatments. It costs about $350,000, on average, to die of cancer in the USA.

By contrast, an American cancer patient can go to Germany for a three week course of treatment for the price of a Honda compact car. What if someone can't afford health insurance? How could he or she possibly afford a six-figure medical bill? Who has a quarter of a million dollars or more just sitting in their bank account?

Natural and effective cancer treatments

The third reason Americans go to Germany for cancer treatment is because they prefer the mild but effective treatments available there. One of the things that surprised most of the American patients is that none of the clinics looked or smelled like a hospital. Rather, the atmosphere was cheerful, friendly, and warm. The German clinics seemed more like hotels or bed & breakfasts. Patients wear their own clothes at the German clinics—not those flimsy hospital gowns that leave your backside exposed.

All German cancer clinics will change your diet. Detoxification, fresh juice and a organic raw food diet is nearly applied in every successful treatment. Exercise and stress reduction is always applied. All the German clinics understand the importance of colonic hydrotherapy, something you can do in the privacy of your home.

The world's best cancer treatment!

You can get it, but thanks to the FTC, FDA and the ACS not in America. So if you live in America, and you are pure, you may be thanking them and the government for your unnecessary suffering and much too early death!—I fear the government will make it even worse! Even harder to be treated with natural cures for cancer in the US—but as I said:" It is just my opinion—But I may be right!™"

Gesundheitszentrum Schmargendorf

The best and most effective all natural treatment for cancer that you can get in Europe is at the c/o Gesundheitszentrum Schmargendorf.

Director Dr. Thomas Hohn MD NMD is not only my colleague and licensed in IBMS Therapy™, he is my master student and took over my patients and health centers from me when I left Germany. He is the most competent healer and MD I ever had the honor to train and to work with together with my most adored friend and student Dr. Holger Crone MD ND HD. Dr. Hohn has had his own TV show: "Naturally Healthy" for over 10 years and is a multi bestselling author and one of the most trusted Medical Doctors in the world. If you want the best therapy by a licensed Medical Doctor that is trained and Licensed in my IBMS-Therapy™ then you need to contact Dr. Hohn in Germany:

Dr. Thomas Hohn MD NMD
Breitestrasse 12
14199 Berlin
Phone-No. 1: 01149 - 30 (Berlin) - 823 50 86 (VIP-Line)
Phone-No. 2: 01149 172 (Vodafone) - 319 10 90 (Cell-Phone) use only in extreme emergencies
Dr. med. Thomas Höhn

Facharzt für Allgemeinmedizin, Naturheilverfahren, Sportmedizin
You have to tell him (or his nurses) that Dr. Leonard Coldwell did send you or you will not get an appointment before the next 18 months or so.

Dr. Hohn is usually booked one to two years in advance but will hold spots for cancer patients in need.

www.goodlifefoundation.com

The Hufeland Klinik in Bad Mergentheim

The medical pioneer who founded the Hufeland Klinik in 1985 was Dr. Wolfgang Woeppel. This is how he expressed his view of cancer: "The tumor is only the late-stage symptom of cancer, which is from the beginning a systemic disease caused by the impaired working of the body's own defense and repair mechanisms. Cancer is not merely the disorder of one organ but is an expression of a comprehensive disorder of the whole person in his or her unity of body and soul. Traditional European naturopathy, empirical medicine, and conventional scientific medicine can be selectively used in a unique way that rebuilds people instead of destroying them."

Dr. Demuth the director states says magnetic-field therapy is one solution. Because magnetic-field therapy promotes circulation and oxygenation, patients have reported improvement with a variety of conditions, including:

- Arthritis
- High blood pressure
- Diabetes
- Stress
- Thyroid conditions
- Skin problems
- Asthma
- Ulcers
- A.D.H.D.
- M.S.
- Cancer

Every town in Germany that has the 3 letters Bad in front of it is a spa or healing town because it has healing water wells or springs that the public has free access too.

Bad or Spa towns feature naturally mineralized waters that people who seek healing can soak in or drink. The water in each well (*quelle in German*) boasts its own unique mineral composition.

Contact information:

Hufeland Klinik

Löffelstelzer Straße 1-3

("ß" is the German symbol for "ss.")

D-97980 Bad Mergentheim, Germany

Contact: Dr. Andreas M. Demuth

Website: http://www.hufeland.com (click on the icon of the British flag for English)

e-mail: info@hufeland.com

phone: 011-49-7931-536-0

fax: 011-49-7931-818-5

BioMed Klinik in Bad Bergzabern

Most of the foreign cancer patients have been told their cancer was "hopeless" and "terminal." Doctors back home have told them, "Nothing more can be done." But BioMed doctors tell them, "We'll try." And BioMed's impressive results prove that those conventional doctors are often wrong.

BioMed is the largest hyperthermia center in Europe, perhaps in the world. But not for long. Like in all of the other German cancer clinics BioMed often uses hyperthermia in conjunction with other therapies.

- A healthful low-meat diet emphasizing fruits and vegetables and discouraging sugar

- Detoxification, including colonic hydrotherapy

- Magnetic-field therapy
- Oxygen therapy
- Ozone therapy
- Hyperthermia (which the receptionist Marit called "fever therapy")
- Dendritic cells
- Psychological counseling and relaxation exercises
- Therapeutic massage
- Qigong (pronounced chee gong) exercises that relieve pain
- Mistletoe therapy
- Insulin potentiation therapy (IPT)
- Infrared therapy for skin metastasis
- Light therapy
- Art therapy
- Music therapy

Contact information:
BioMed Klinik
Rischberger Straße 5 + 8
D-76887 Bad Bergzabern, Germany
Head physician:
Dr. Dieter Hager, M.D., Ph.D., D.Sc.
Contact: Marit Ehnert
Website: www.biomed-klinik.de
e-mail: medinfo@biomed-klinik.de
Phone: 011-49-6343-705-0
Fax: 011-49-6343-705-913

Klinik Marinus am Stein in Brannenburg

A surgeon who recommends against cancer surgery, Dr. Axel Weber, M.D., is this historic motto of the entire medical profession: *Primum non nocere*! The English translation for this Latin motto is: First do no harm! Why should a patient have surgery if there's a better way to get rid of the cancer?

Here are some of the therapies the clinic offers:

*   Whole-body hyperthermia with low-dose chemo

*   Local hyperthermia

*   Magnetic-field therapy

*   Detoxification procedures including the foot bath detox

*   Oxygen therapy

*   Ozone therapy

*   Mistletoe therapy

*   Intravenous vitamin C and selenium

*   Foot reflexology

*   Electro-dermal screening (a non-invasive diagnostic technique using acupressure points)

*   Acupuncture

Like the other German cancer clinics, Klinik Marinus recommends that patients eat plenty of fruits and vegetables, cut down on meat, and avoid sugar. The clinic includes a room where Dr. Weber occasionally performs small surgeries when necessary. He performs no major surgeries or abdominal surgeries.

Why surgery fails to eliminate cancer

"It's better for the patient to avoid surgery if at all possible. As a surgeon, he usually recommend *against* surgery. Unless you get at the *cause* of the cancer, you'll get metastasis. It's not enough just to get rid of the tumor. You have to get rid of the metastasized cells, and that requires treating the whole body."

Without a doubt, Dr. Weber is an expert in hyperthermia, an important part of the whole treatment plan. Ten years ago he founded the Hyperthermia Society of Germany, and he's given 14,000 hyperthermia treatments since then.

Contact information:

Klinik Marinus am Stein

Biberstraße 30

83098 Brannenburg, Germany

Contact: Dr. Axel Weber

Website: www.klinik-marinus.de (The clinic is in the process of creating an English website, which might or might not be online by the time you read this.)

e-mail: info@klinik-marinus.de

Phone: 011-49-8034-908-0

Fax: 011-49-8034-908-299

Dr. Alexander Herzog's Fachklinik in Bad Salzhausen (Nidda, near Frankfurt)

Dr. Herzog is a grand master of hyperthermia. There are three kinds of whole-body hyperthermia: Moderate hyperthermia, in which the patient's core temperature is raised to 101-103 degrees Fahrenheit for two hours, which simulates a natural fever.

Systemic hyperthermia, which raises the core temperature to 105 degrees F. Extreme hyperthermia, which goes up to 107 degrees F. But Dr. Herzog is one of the few physicians in the world with the equipment, training, and experience to use all three kinds of hyperthermia.

Contact information:

Fachklinik Dr. Herzog

(Specialty Hospital Dr. Herzog)

Kurstraße 16-18

D-63667 Nidda, Germany

Contact: Dr. A. Herzog

Website: www.fachklinikdrherzog.de

e-mail: info@hospitaldrherzog.de

Phone: 011-49-6043-983-0

Fax: 011-49-6043-983-194

Pro Leben Klinik in Igls/Innsbruck, Austria

How a Siberian medicine man cures cancer with snake venom!

Dr. Daudert tells an amazing story about a medicine man he met in an isolated corner of the Siberian wilderness. This area is so remote there's no physician within a 250-mile radius, so the villagers all depended on the medicine man for their health. A woman came to him with a large, ugly tumor of the breast. The medicine man let Dr. Daudert examine his patient. The cancer was obviously severe. The woman had no money to take the train to Moscow for treatment in a cancer clinic there. She had only the medicine man to help her. She put her life in his hands.

The medicine man told her, "No problem." And then he left. His wife told Dr. Daudert, "He's looking for a snake. He needs the venom." He came back with a poisonous snake, from which he milked the venom. Then he mixed the fresh venom with raw honey and covered the tumor with a poultice made from the venom/ honey mixture. Just three days later the tumor had shrunk by 20 percent! The woman was happy. Her pain was gone!

Doctors at the University of Moscow heard about the effectiveness of the medicine man's cancer cure and are now studying snake venom for its medicinal value. While other Russian industries have their share of problems, Dr. Daudert explains that there's no "pharmaceutical mafia" in Russia to hamper, discourage, or discredit such research into natural medicines.

Dr. Daudert runs tests that show that *no* chemotherapy whatsoever will be helpful for patients. He says, "Doctors are blindly giving chemotherapy to some patients while the cancer cells smile and the patients die."

Some years ago I had a vet that cured one of my horses with an inoperable tumor on its colon exit with spider venom that he injected and 2 days later the horse was cured.

Colonic hydrotherapy and coffee enemas the basic treatment for cancer patients.

According to Dr. Daudert, colonic hydrotherapy is "very important." Indeed, all the German physicians we interviewed agreed foursquare on the importance of colonic hydrotherapy.

A gunked-up gut goes with disease. A clean, efficiently functioning colon goes with health.

Dr. Daudert says colonic hydrotherapy is so important that he teaches the patients how to do it at home and keep up their colonics. Another important tool at Pro Leben is the darkfield microscope—an amazing diagnostic tool that magnifies the patient's *living* blood 14,000 times. This microscope enables a trained doctor to see what's *really* going on with the patient's health. Pro Leben employs a Russian doctor who's a master of darkfield microscopy. Personally I always added coffee enemas to my treatment protocol for all cancer patients.

Contact information for Dr. Daudert's Pro
Leben Klinik in Igls/Innsbruck, Austria:
Pro Leben Klinik
Hilberstraße 3
A—6080 Igls/Innsbruck, Austria
Contact: Dr. Frank Daudert
Website: www.prolebenklinik-igls.at
e-mail: office@prolebenklinik-igls.at
Phone: 011-43-5123-798-620
Fax: 011-43-5123-798-625
Leonardis Klinik in Bad Heilbrunn

Leonardis Klinik is in the Bavarian Alps
Orthodox cancer treatment is like "deforestation"
Leonardis uses a therapy called "photopheresis," which we didn't see at any of the other clinics. It's a procedure in which the clinic draws about 10 or 15 milliliters of blood from the patient, mixes it with an herb, St. John's Wort, and rein-fuses and activates it through ultraviolet light. Dr. Draczynski explained that this therapy boosts the natural killer cells.

The treatment takes about 30 to 45 minutes. A couple of therapies were missing at Leonardis: magnetic-field therapy and colonic hydrotherapy. But unlike whole-body hyperthermia, which requires a machine costing over a quarter of a million dollars, magnetic-field therapy and colonic hydrotherapy are affordable so you can do them in the privacy of your home.

Colonic hydrotherapy a powerful tool
Giving patients coffee enemas always helps. The benefits of coffee enemas against cancer are well established in the medical literature.

And when the coffee is administered rectally, it goes directly to the patient's liver and stimulates it to flush out toxins. This liver-flushing action also helps the fight against cancer. The Leonardis clinic uses both local hyperthermia and whole-body hyperthermia.

Before whole-body hyperthermia, the patient is pre-heated in a warm tub for 15 or 20 minutes. Then the patient goes into the hyperthermia tent. Dr. Draczynski said Leonardis uses moderate whole-body hyperthermia, taking the patient's body temperature up to 39 degrees Celsius, about 102.2 degrees Fahrenheit. For whole-body hyperthermia, this temperature plateau is low compared to those in some other clinics we visited.

The powerful therapy that outsmarts cancer cells isn't available in U.S.

Cancer cells can cleverly hide from the patient's immune system. One therapy that can outsmart the cancer cells is dendritic cell vaccines. Dr. Draczynski's clinic uses this therapy.

Of course, thanks to the FTC and FDA Dendritic cell therapy isn't yet available in America.

Contact information:

Leonardis Klinik

Abt-Walther-Weg 14-16

83670 Bad Heilbrunn, Germany

Contact: Mr. Rudolphi

Website: www.leonardis-klinik.de

e-mail: info@leonardis-klinik.de

Phone: 011-49-8046-187-0

Fax: 011-49-8046-187-10

How To Find The Right Treatment For You

If you are not sure which cancer clinic is right for you, please write and I or my staff will help you. Go to www.InstinctBasedMedicine.com

You can also get treated by my certified IBMS™ Therapists and practitioners that are all licensed MDs, NDs, HDs or NMDs and trained personally by me.

Share Your Stories!

If you have a story about the medical system, your doctor or what they did to you or people you know or love, please send it to me and we will publish these stories without the names. However, you will need to give me the names confidentially for legal reasons, though I will not disclose them. Write to InstinctBasedMedicine@gmail.com

For free medical advice write to my colleague and master student Dr. Thomas Hohn MD NMD DrHohn@goodlifefoundation.com

If you are able to read German see *The Cholesterol Lie* by my German colleague medical Professor and MD Walter Hartenbach. It will blow your mind.

Fulfilling a Lifelong Dream

As you probably know, I am working on the realization of my lifelong dream to create the largest and most complex health resort in the world. All forms of therapy will be in one single place, up to 1000 acres. There will not be any reason for patients, no matter what their goal is, to go anywhere else. We will also have a natural dentist, beauticians and more so that even if people just want to get recharged and regenerated they can do so.

We are also building a community in that place where people can buy homes and live in a safe and health-oriented community where everything is organic and natural and everybody is like-minded and positive.

Please write me or just subscribe to my free newsletter and you will be informed of our progress. www.InstinctBasedMedicine.com

I Would Cure Everyone For Free If I Legally Would Be Allowed To Do So

If there was ever the possibility that I could apply my entire IBMS™ without any restrictions legally in the USA, I would treat everybody that bought my books and the IBMS™ series, and those who helped me to achieve the goal of legally applying my IBMS™ in the US, for free.

Help me to make sure that we get an amendment to the constitution for health freedom and patient rights. If you want to donate to my legal defense and research foundation so that I can fight off all of the legal attacks they will come up with to stop my messages of fast, simple and safe natural cures for cancer and all other health challenges, please send your check in any amount to:

Dr. Leonard Coldwell, Legal Research Found,

1150 Hungryneck Blvd Suite C 379

Mount Pleasant, South Carolina 29464

Thank you for your help and support. It's people like you, the health freedom fighters of this world, which can make my goal in life attainable; to help educate everyone on how to cure their own personal cancer and to avoid the slaughter of the medical community!

"Stand up together with me to fight for an amendment to the constitution of the United States of America, for: Health Freedom and Patient Rights! And all the evil in the medical profession will disappear on its own!"

A Note in Closing

Please remember that I do not believe in physical cures of cancer or any other terminal diseases, for that matter. I believe cancer does not even exist as an illness. If we are out of energetic balance—which is always the result of mental and emotional stress—we create a perfect environment for cancer to grow.

Some basic treatments, mainly detoxification and supplemental alkalization of the body, are important and can speed up the healing process dramatically. Health means 100% optimum function of all body systems, as well as 100% of mental and emotional health. You are healthy or you are not, there is nothing in the middle. After all, you cannot be a little bit pregnant! So, you cannot be a little bit healthy or a little bit sick. You are healthy or you are not.

Let me say at this point that I don't believe you should be a fanatic or radical in healthy behavior. In my experience, if you do 70% of the right things, you can do 30% of the wrong things if you are healthy and nothing bad will happen as long as you use common sense and my IBMS™ to repair, detoxify and regenerate on a regular basis.

Most of all, if you don't feel right or are sick, you have to do the right thing 100% of the time until you're healed again. Keep in mind everything that I have told you about in this book and in my book Instinct Based Medicine How to Survive Your Illness And Your Doctor. www.InstinctBasedMedicine.com

And again: I believe that only chronic mental and emotional stress can cause terminal diseases like cancer. I cannot stress this enough! Please get my IBMS™ stress reduction system™ or my IBMS-Life-Therapy™ or the IBMS™ Library of Life™ session which will help you with every possible life challenge.

If you have any questions please don't hesitate to write me at InstinctBasedMedicine@gmail.com or get individual free medical health advice from my master student Dr. Thomas Hohn MD NMD and write him at DrHohn@goodlifefoundation.com

Thank you for reading my book. I strongly believe if you have read the entire book that you are a winner, a self-healer, a doer and not a quitter! I believe in you and your powers to heal yourself.

There is no healing force outside the human body—you are the only person that can make you sick and the only person that can cure you. If you apply all the things you learned from me in my book or books and CD sessions you will be able to find, create and apply your individual personal solution: Your only answer to Cancer!

I say goodbye for now my dear friend and I hope I could open your mind for the truth: That none that makes money on your pain, suffering, symptoms, illness and death can have your best interest in mind! Therefore you have to take charge and responsibility for your own health and life and that of your children and loved ones. Never ever give the power over your health and life decisions over to someone else! It is your life and you are the only person that has to live with the consequences of your decisions and not the ones with the "good" suggestions. Therefore get educated and study: health, happiness, vitality and life to be able to make your own sophisticated decisions for your own life and that of your children.

I hope you could learn through my book, that **if you are diagnosed with cancer** or any other so called incurable disease—that **you do not have to die**! Cancer is naturally curable, and so is, in my experience and opinion, every other disease or condition. Just make sure you don't allow the government to interfere or control our health and treatment choices. Vote everybody out of office that does not support health freedom and the Constitution! Have hope. Stay strong and have a long, happy, successful and healthy life!

If you have any questions or suggestions please write to
instinctbasedmedicine@gmail.com
or go to
www.instinctbasedmedicine.com

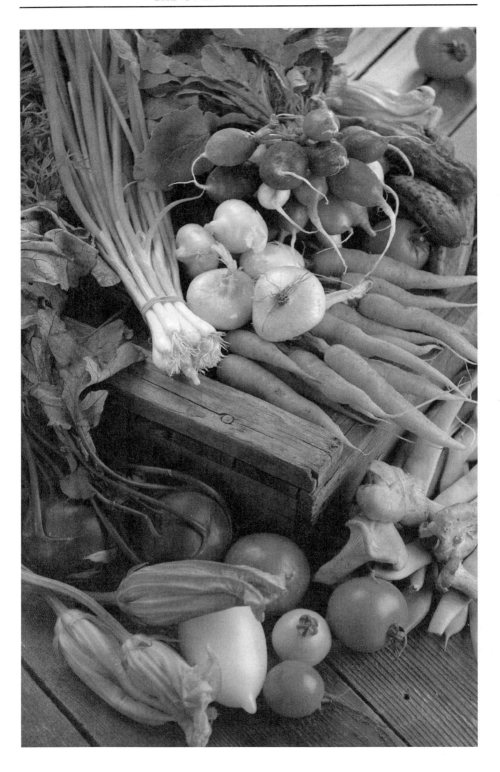

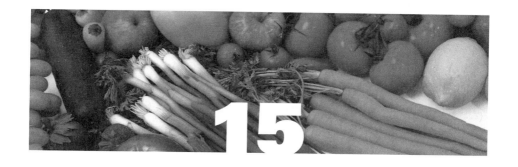

ORGANIC WHOLE FOOD

Organic whole food is instructed by the Bible and Christian stress reduction and Healing Prayer CD's.

The inspiration for Phi Plus, originally came from what is referred to as Pulse in the King James Version of the Bible, from the Old Testament, in the Book of Daniel 1:12 & 16.

1:12 Prove thy servants, I beseech thee, ten days; and let them give us pulse to eat, and water to drink.

1:16 Thus Melzar took away the portion of their meat, and the wine that they should drink; and gave them pulse.

My friend Dan Allen, his wife and a friend were on a water and juice fast in the late 1980's at Mt. Lassen in Northern California.

As Dan was reading the Book of Daniel in the Old Testament he recognized the power of Pulse and water. In Chapter one, Daniel and his three friends ate only Pulse and drank only water for 10 days, rather than the King's rich food and wine. At the end of the 10 days, Daniel and his friends proved to be stronger and healthier than all the men. They stayed on the diet permanently. And in all matters of wisdom and understanding, that the king inquired of them, he found them ten times better than all the magicians and astrologers that were in all his realm.

This inspired Dan to create a recipe of what Pulse may have been and PHI Plus is one such creation. Since the recipe of Pulse is unknown, only that it was a vegetarian combination, PHI Plus is a combination of all natural organic whole food ingredients including nuts, seeds, grains, fruits, vegetables, berries, herbs, oils and spices.

Now, thanks to The Wholefood Farmacy, you too can experience a remarkable difference in your health and how you feel, which will also be observed by others. The Wholefood Farmacy has put together several 7 & 13 or 14 Day Nutritional Events which make it possible for anyone to experience what Daniel and his three friends did. After Nutritional Events some of our customer's have reported benefits of higher levels of energy, improved overall vitality, safe and effective weight management, increased mental alertness, improved function of digestion and elimination with a strengthened immune system. These Nutritional events are made up of nutrient-dense raw whole foods, including Phi Plus, that are formulated with ingredients as close to nature as possible. Eating these foods gives your body the nutrients it wants, needs, understands, and knows how to utilize at the cellular level. Plus, as you enjoy one of the Nutritional Events, consisting of wonderful foods from 'nature's table', you will also be replacing, or eliminating, foods which actually may be toxic to your body, just as Daniel and his friends did! We all use Dr. Leonard Coldwell's new Stress Reduction and Health Prayer CD set for Christians! It brings us closer to God. See www.instinctbasedmedicine.com and look for: **Quiet Time!**

Steven Lowell Tilton
www.greatwholefood.com
President/CEO
The Wholefood Farmacy
423-921-7848
"Let thy food be thy medicine, medicine be thy food"
~Hippocrates 460-370 BC

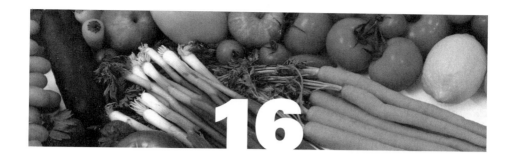

DIET FOR A HEALTHY PLANET

John Eagle Freedom's dream is to unite the parents of the world by revealing the truths that Dr. Leonard Coldwell shares in his book. John's personal journey to health was accomplished when he took responsibility for his own immune system. "How can you fix a problem if you're not aware of the problem?" He says. John believes Americans are too close to the forest and their taste buds that they can't see the trees nor can they see the cause of their sicknesses and diseases. They've been deceived by the media, medical profession and corporate America that healing comes from outside of the body with magic pills and surgery. John knows that all healing begins by enhancing our own immune system, by practicing the natural health laws. Proper hydration with proper drinking protocol, exercise, sunlight, proper breathing, proper nutrition, mineralization, and enzymes, all are a part of healthy living.

John found out he was a diabetic at 60 with a blood sugar-level over 500. One day he was traveling down the highway at 65 miles an hour when he had a blood sugar black-out rolling his automobile. That was his wake-up call. John believed that he was healthy, he had a big belly, good strength for his age, and energy. He educated himself about the miraculous healing nature life-force that lies within the human body. In a very short time he had a better body than when he was 19. Then he had an encounter with an 18-wheeler, not once, but twice! He had over $300,000.00 worth of medical bills, with both rotator cuffs shattered, and five vertebrae in his neck and back blown out. Doctors said to him, "John, let us operate on you or choose the color of wheel chair, because you'll be in it the rest of your life." He replied, "I'm going to give my Master Healer a chance first!" His healing journey began with physical therapy 5 days a week, 3 surgeries on his shoulders, still having 50 seizures a day, with only 35-40 % range of motion after two years, and memory failure (he had to number his grandchildren, 1-10). Then, after two years, his doctors said, "John, you didn't get it in two years, you're not going to get it."

That's when his friends sent him to Hippocrates. John asked Brian Clement, the director, "Why couldn't I heal, being a raw-foodist?" Brian's response, "That's your problem, John, you need to be a living-foodist." A living foodist only eats raw foods in their highest enzymatic state that are uncooked. John spent 4 months at Hippocrates, he recovered his full range of motion, seizures stopped, and his memory returned. His blood-sugar returned to normal, impotency from high-blood pressure, cirrhosis of the liver, due to life-style—all gone! John now has the liver of an athlete!

The journey of 1,000 miles, we've all heard, begins with the first step. John says, "The journey begins with the thought of the journey." How can we begin the journey of health if we're not aware that we're sick? Do we have to wait until death looks us in the eye? It's very difficult to kick an addiction, whether it is alcoholism, nicotine, caffeine, sexual, and gambling, etc. People do not see that addiction to junk food, over-processed food, cooked food, soda pop, sugar, etc. is a problem. Being in denial never eliminates a problem and we, the people of America have a problem; we are facing the largest economical tsunami, the world has ever faced! We have a health care budget approaching $3 Trillion, 95% of which is spent the last 30 days of a person's life. Corporate America, pharmaceutical, the medical profession, and we the people are responsible. By taking responsibility for our own health by educating and putting into practice simple, natural health laws, we can once again be a healthy nation.

John's vision, HEALTH CITY U.S.A., began in Southwestern Missouri, Springfield/Branson, better known as the buckle on the Bible belt. Dr. George Malkmus asks the question, "Why do Christians and non-Christian get sick at the same rate?" His answer, "...because they eat at the same trough!" John and his friends agree. John and his author friends, are committed and have joined together to produce the first book, The Healing Nature of Jesus. John has a vision of placing this book, and other books written by the contributing health expert authors, in the hands of every minister and church that has ears to hear, and eyes to see beginning in this area and then taking it to the world, encouraging not only themselves but also the flocks under their care. Doing this will directly impact the proper care and feeding of the children of the world.

John is also a global health summit leader of which there are 23 recognized in the world who meet every two years at Hippocrates Health Clinic, in West Palm Beach, Florida. These leaders participate in a symposium to discuss the ultimate diet for vibrant health and longevity.

The ultimate diet to look good, feel great and thrive is revealed in Diana Store's book, *Raw Food Works*.

The Health Summit leaders from eight countries (with a combined total of 434 years following this lifestyle) support the following standards:

The Optimum Diet for Health/Longevity:

- Vegan (no animal products of any kind, cooked or raw)

- Organic

- Whole Foods

- High in nutrition such as vitamins, antioxidants, and phytonutrients

- Highly mineralized

- Contains a significant quantity of chlorophyll-rich green foods

- Contains adequate complete protein from plant sources

- Contains a large proportion of high-water-content foods

- Provides excellent hydration

- Includes raw vegetable juices

- Contains all essential fatty acids, including Omega-3 fatty acids from naturally occurring plant sources

- Is at lest 80% raw (the remaining to be Vegan, whole food, and organic)

- Has moderate yet adequate caloric intake

- Contains only low to moderate sugar and exclusively from whole-food sources (fruitarianism is strongly discouraged)

- Contains adequate amounts of unprocessed salts, as needed (depending upon your constitution)

- Is nutritionally optimal for both detoxification and rebuilding

We also agree that:

- Deficiency of Vitamin B-12 is a global issue for mental and physical health, for *anyone on any* diet. Therefore, supplementation with Vitamin B-12 is advised.

- The addition of enzyme-active substances *(even in their raw form)*, such as cocoa/chocolate, coffee, caffeinated teas, and alcohol are highly discouraged.

- This way of eating can be further optimized by tailoring it based on *individual needs* (within the principles stated).

- Benefits derived by following these are proportional to how well they are followed.

- We will remain open-minded, and this information will be updated and expanded upon if necessary, as new research becomes available.

- Diet is a critical part of a healthy lifestyle, yet not the entire picture. A full-spectrum, health-supportive lifestyle is encouraged. This includes physical exercise, exposure to sunshine, as well as psychological health. Avoiding environmental toxins and toxic products is essential. Paramount is pure water (for consumption and bathing,) the use of natural fiber clothing, and non-toxic personal-care products. Also consider healthy options in home furnishings/building materials and related items.

All participating leaders agree that eating according to the International Living Food Summit Guidelines will significantly address the urgent issues of health, environmental sustainability, world hunger, and a compassionate respect for life.

John and his friends are doing everything that they can do to reveal the TRUTH to the world! They ask that you join them and do your part. Ask your ministers to receive the gifts they offer in LOVE and share the TRUTH with their congregations: it is the life-force placed in out temples by our creator, and enhanced by obedience by treating the body as a temple and not a trash can. We can return to the vibrant health of our youth. Enjoy Heaven here on earth by eliminating all pain, sickness and disease, and enjoy the journey of life, and experience True Love by loving yourself first. Join us and be responsible for your own immune system. It's not the food in our life—the life in our food!

John and his friend Viktoras Kulvinskas—better known as the grandfather of the living food movement—requests you to get behind Dr. Leonard Coldwell and the global summit leaders who speak the TRUTH on your behalf forming ranks on the front lines. We are willing to put our lives honor and financial future at risk, the same way the founding fathers got behind the TRUTH of the Declaration of Independence and the Constitution of the United States of America. Dr. Leonard Coldwell has a plan by creating an amendment to the Constitution, that we have a right to health in America. We the people have the power! The time has come—let Freedom ring all over the United States of America!

The following leaders support the optimum diet for a healthy planet:
(listed in alphabetical order)

Fred Bisci, PhD – USA

Tamera Campbell – Vision – USA

Rajaa Chbani – Pharmacie L'Unite – Morocco

Marie Christine; Lhermitte Chemin du mas Magnuel – France

Katherine Clark, RN, CMT, MSU – USA

Anna Maria Clement, CN,NMD, PhD – Hippocrates Health Institute – USA

Brian Clement, CN, NMD, PhD – Hippocrates Health Institute –USA

Gabriel Cousens, MD, MD(H) – Diplomat American Board of Holistic Medicine – USA

Brenda Cobb – Living Foods Institute – USA

Carole Dougoud – Institute Haute Vitalite – Switzerland

Dorit – Serenity Spaces – USA

Kare Engstrom – Dietician – Sweden

John Eagle Freedom - Healing Nature Press, Health City USA, Vibrant Life, The Hour of Truth – USA

Viktoras Kulvinskas – "Grandfather" of the Living Foods Movement – USA

Dan Ladermann – Living Light International – USA

George Malkmus – Hallelujah Acres – USA

Rhonda Malkmus – Hallelujah Acres – USA

Paul Nison – The Raw Life – USA

Katrina Rainoshek – Juice Feasting – USA

David Rainoshek – Juice Feasting – USA

Claudine Richard – Naturopath – France

Michael Saiber – Vision – USA

Cherie Soria – Living Light International – USA

Jameth Sheridan, ND – HealthForce Nutritionals – USA

Diana Store – Raw Superfoods – UK/The Netherlands

Jill Swyers – Living Foods For Health – UK/Portugal

Walter J. Urban, PhD – USA – Costa Rica

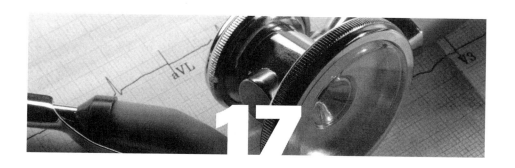

ENZYMES: THE FOUNDATION FOR WELLNESS

Viktoras Kulvinskas, MS

Adequate cellular nutrition is dependent on a combination of factors: dietary choices, method of food preparation, degree of thorough chewing, as well as the body's functional efficiency in digesting and assimilating food. Eating food-based enzymes is a key to helping your body maximize your genetic potential, even if you sometimes choose less-than optimal lifestyle habits. Using plant-based enzymes increases the availability of nutrients to the billions of cells that are your physical body. Your choosing to "dine with enzymes" can mean the difference between a life of mediocre or marginal health, and the experience of high-level wellness and abundant energy.

What are enzymes?
The word "enzyme" comes from the Greek word *enzymas*, which means "to ferment" or "cause a change." Enzymes are the foundation for all cell regeneration. They play a key role in the transformation of undigested food into the nutrients that are absorbed on the cellular level. With

proper nutrition, we have the energy to participate in the dance of the living. An enzyme is a specialized protein structure that carries with it an energetic charge. Enzymes speed up chemical reactions that normally take place very slowly or not at all. It is the energy behind the protein structure that makes enzymes different from other protein-based substances. It is the energetic life principle, sometimes called *prana*, or chi, that animates all life forms. The father of modern enzyme therapy, Dr. Edward Howell, once said that enzymes emit a "kind of radiation" that can be picked up on Kirlian photographs. Howell can be singled out from other researchers because he stressed that enzymes are not merely expendable, protein-based chemical catalysts that move along chemical reactions. He forcefully argued that enzymes are none other than units of life-energy that use various protein molecules as their carriers.

Enzymes are much more sensitive to destruction by heat or cold than vitamins and minerals. Food cooked over 118 degrees F for more than a half an hour will kill all naturally-occurring enzymes. In the event that dry heat is used, the critical temperature for enzyme destruction is about 150 F. Enzymes are the true workers in and out of our cells. As Dr. Richard Gerber MD states, "the enzymes catalyze specific reactions of chemicals either to create structure through molecular assemblies or to provide the electrochemical fire to run the cellular engines and ultimately keep the entire system working."

There are thousands of different enzymes, so many that one cannot separate enzyme activity with the process of life itself. From moving a muscle to blinking an eye, no biological work can be accomplished independent of enzymes. Without enzymes, the body would be nothing but inorganic matter.

Types of enzymes

Enzymes can be grouped into three main categories. The first category consists of the digestive enzymes, which the digestive system collects, manufactures and secretes to break down food. Examples of digestive enzymes are protease, which digests protein; amylase, which digests starch; and lipase, which digests fat. Each enzyme almost always has only one specific function that it carries out. For example, the enzyme protease only digests protein. The enzyme amylase only digests starches.

The second type of enzymes is composed of metabolic enzymes, which are present in every cell, tissue, and organ and act as biochemical catalysts in the second-to-second functioning of living cells. The metabolic antioxidant enzyme superoxide dismutase (SOD), which is present in all cells, reduces free radical damage, and thus retards the aging process. Raw foods, especially sprouts and algae, are rich in SOD.

The third class of enzymes is made up of various food enzymes, which come from raw, uncooked foods. The process of enzymatic digestion begins when you masticate your food in your mouth. When you chew, you not only mix the enzyme ptyalin from your salivary glands into the food, but allow the food-based enzymes present in the food to be released onto itself. This occurs from the moment that you rupture the cell walls of the food with your teeth.

Most fresh, well-grown produce has at least enough enzymes to digest the specific amount of protein, starch or fat found in the food itself. As a general rule, the higher the caloric content of an uncooked food, the more enzymes Nature will have put into the food to handle the exact amount of nutrients present. Nature is so considerate and thoughtful, don't you think? So, foods high in protein will have a high amount of protease or protein-digesting enzyme. Examples are blue-green algae and sunflower seeds. Foods such as whole oats have a high amount of amylase or starch-digesting enzymes. Foods such as avocados and nuts have naturally-occurring lipase or fat-digesting enzymes. Nature is so balanced—I wish I could balance my checkbook as easily.

One of the myths still held by many health food consumers is that eating a raw vegetable salad alongside an otherwise cooked meal is sufficient to digest the cooked food portion of the meal. The reality of the situation is that since here is a direct correlation between the number of calories in a food and the amount of enzymes present, low-calorie salads have relatively few enzymes to help out in digesting any other food you may be eating. Unless the salad is composed of sprouts (which are naturally high in enzymes because they are young plants), you cannot count on raw salads to be of much help in digesting other foods.

Enzyme Logic in dollars and sense

Let's play a little with the concept of enzymes by using our day-to-day experience of banking as a metaphor. Your body's enzymes can be likened to cash reserves in your own life-force bank account. Each time you eat enzyme-less food, you tax your system by making a withdrawal from this enzyme bank. Meal by meal you decrease your enzyme net worth, which can be equated with your life potential. Since at least half of all enzyme capital in the body is assigned to digesting foods, eating life-less cooked foods in effect puts a continual hold on 50% of your budget. Your individual budget limit is determined by your genetic inheritance.

If one's enzyme capital is frozen in this way, your ability to allocate funds to improve the quality of your life is then on hold to the tune of 50% of your net worth! You'll then have limited enzyme resources with which to make much-needed home improvements (cleansing and re-building organs and tissues) and protecting your enzyme life savings via a strong immune system. To complicate matters, your bills are coming due, and guess what, your account is low in funds! You're desperate, so you borrow (take stimulants such as coffee to keep going) because your credit rating (overall health) is bad, due to years and years of withdrawals. You now wish that you had made more enzyme deposits in your life-force bank account, so that you wouldn't be finding yourself in arrears, experiencing energy deficiencies. Now that you know how health finances work, start investing in your future health by taking plant-based enzymes today, before life hands you a bill that you can't afford to pay! It could be the best investment, with a return of new youthful energy and freedom from some of the crises of middle age.

Enzymes throughout history

In the 1890s, the forerunners of the modern science of nutrition discovered building-block substances in food. They named these building-blocks *proteins*. At the turn of the 20th century, a new word was coined to refer to a class of food-based, bio-active, organically-bound chemical substances found to be essential for human health. These substances were called *vitamins*. And about a decade or so later, the importance of organic *minerals* in food was recognized to be equally essential to health.

More than 100 years after the birth of modern scientific nutrition, we find ourselves at an exciting juncture. A missing link in our understanding of the life-giving properties of food is being illuminated by the increasing acceptance of the critical role of food-based enzymes for health and longevity. I think that in the near future, the recognition of the impact of enzymes on health will have even more profound repercussions than many of the discoveries related to vitamins, minerals, and proteins have had.

We can begin a discussion of nutrition as it relates to enzymes by talking about our first food: milk. Numerous medical studies and current public health statistics confirm what our prehistoric ancestors knew, that infants who were breast-fed on human mother's milk had fewer health problems than those infants who were raised on pasteurized cow's milk. Aside from the self-evident fact that human mother's milk is ideally suited for human infants and cow's milk is ideally suited for calves, it is significant that the former is unheated and therefore enzyme-rich and the latter is heated and therefore enzyme-poor.

More than 20 years ago, I discovered Dr. Howell's long out-of-print first book gathering dust in the basement of a medical library where I was doing health research. Published in 1939, this limited edition book was entitled, *The Status of Food Enzymes in Digestion and Metabolism*. With much effort I traced its author, who was in his 80s, and found him affiliated with an enzyme manufacturing company he himself had founded in the 1930s. Dr. Howell graciously gave me permission to reprint and update the book under the new title, *Food Enzymes for Health and Longevity*. About a decade later, Howell's classic was again republished in a simplified and popularized version by Avery Press and renamed *Enzyme Nutrition*. With this last release, the long-ignored discoveries of Dr. Howell spread to many health practitioners and seekers of health around the world.

Dr. Howell's food enzyme concept

Dr. Edward Howell was the first nutritional scientist to develop a larger experimental and theoretical body of work aimed at answering the complex and critically important question, "what are the connections between food or supplement-based enzyme intake, health, disease, and longevity?" Howell devoted his entire adult life to conducting numerous animal and human experiments in his attempt to strengthen the theory that food enzyme deficiencies promote disease and premature aging, whereas enzyme-rich diets promote good health and longevity. To this end, his book, *The Status of Food Enzymes in Digestion and Metabolism* cited more than 400 research papers, which in his day represented the cutting edge of science. Modern researchers have yet to comprehend fully the implications of that book. As Dr. Howell once said, "To say that the body can easily digest and assimilate cooked foods may someday prove to be the most grievous oversight yet committed by science."

Dr. Howell theorized that on a largely cooked, low-enzyme diet, the digestive system borrows enzymes from the body's general metabolic enzyme pool to help digest enzyme-less cooked food. Howell emphasized that the consequences of this adaptive measure were great, in that diverting enzymes from one system to another eventually weakened the functioning of these other systems and the body in general. For example, he argued that the immune system was compromised due to gradual enzyme deficiency and that this set the stage for numerous health problems such as allergies, cancer, and diabetes. If he were alive today, Howell would undoubtedly include AIDS on this list.

In treating his patients, Dr. Howell initially prescribed raw food diets but soon found this to be impractical because many patients lacked the willpower required to stay on such a regime. By 1932, however, he had already developed a plant-based enzyme supplement designed to replace the enzymes lost in a typical cooked food diet.

Dr. Howell discovered that enzyme supplements from plant sources were uniquely effective. The following are just a few of some of Howell's basic concepts.

Food enzymes are essential nutrients.

Being more fragile to the effects of heat than vitamins and minerals, food enzymes are destroyed by the high temperature of cooking.

When food is chewed and swallowed in its raw natural state, enzymes immediately go to work in the upper cardiac portion of the stomach.

Eating a low-enzyme, cooked food diet increases the size of the pancreas, a sign that this organ is being overworked. He further hypothesized that this condition is a precursor to various forms of dysfunction such as hypoglycemia, diabetes and metabolic imbalances.

A deficiency of food enzymes in the diet gives rise to "digestive leukocytosis," (excess white cells in the digestive system and blood) which is not the case when raw, high-enzyme foods are eaten.

More than 60 years ago, Dr. Edward Howell began to cultivate one special species of the many aspergillus plants that existed in the plant kingdom. He picked the "oryzae" strain because there were no harmful aflatoxins (a type of poison) associated with this plant. More importantly, however, this strain contained a rich store of the very same enzymes that the human body used to digest food.

For the first time in recorded history, Howell gave the powdered form of these little plants directly to human patients. He found that spergillus orzae was a key to treating a whole host of seemingly unrelated ailments. Because of the success of his clinical work, he dedicated his life to working out a theoretical and experimental platform to explain how these seeming miracles had been accomplished. The development of the "Food Enzyme Concept" in human nutrition was this great man's life's work.

This chapter would not have been written, nor perhaps would I be as alive and healthy as I am today, if it were not for the amazing properties of these "angel-hair-in-appearance" microscopic plants. I have been eating aspergillus plant digestive enzymes for more than 20 years. I have also experimented with other animal and vegetarian-based enzymes such as pancreatin, pepsin, papain and bromelain. I have concluded that aspergillus enzymes are far superior to these other enzyme sources.

Recycling and specificity of enzymes

The editor of the *Scottish Medical Journal* (1966) wrote that "probably nearly half of our daily production of protein in the body are enzymes." In a way, our bodies are like big enzyme factories. There is strong evidence that the body seeks to conserve its digestive enzymes. In the prestigious scientific journal *Science,* Liebow and Rohman (1975) describe an experiment in which it was found that pancreatic enzymes given by mouth can be absorbed intact from the gut, transported through the bloodstream and then be re-secreted into the duodenum by the pancreas. If only my home's heating system were as efficient!

There is an antagonistic relationship between the demands of the digestive system for a continual supply of enzymes and the need of the organs, glands and immune system for enzymes with which to do their work. The competition for enzyme resources can be easily relieved by the consumption of food-source enzymes. Dr. Guyon's authoritative *Textbook of Medical Physiology* (1986) states that the pancreas, stomach and possibly other organs secrete specific digestive enzymes according to the type and quantity of food present. The ingestion of plant enzymes may have been conserving effect on the body's enzyme potential, possibly aiding cell and organ regeneration by digesting the food which normally would have required the body's own pancreatic enzymes.

Co-enzymes make super-enzymes

Organic minerals and vitamins are sometimes bound to enzymes that are integrated into the enzyme structure and are referred to as co-enzymes. According to Dr. Maynard Murray, MD, every naturally occurring organic mineral should be considered essential for optimal health. Minerals are essential for the working of enzymes, and enzymes are essential for the working of minerals. A few examples: if a certain enzyme is lacking an essential co-factor mineral such as zinc, then the enzyme cannot successfully activate vitamin A to do its work.

If a co-factor of vitamin C lacks the proline hydroxylase enzyme, this will lead to impaired collagen synthesis which will profoundly affect muscle recovery and wound healing. Co-enzymes give the enzymes the power to do their work. Medical researcher Dr. Haigivara MD concludes: "Modern science has made it clear that all chemical changes within the cells of humankind are performed by the action of enzymes. It has been found that minerals have much to do with the activities of enzymes. In that sense, minerals can be said to be enzymes for the enzymes."

Enzymes are, without a doubt, the most important and most overlooked elements in nutrition today. A deficiency of merely one enzyme may cause the malfunctioning of an entire metabolic chain reaction in the body, thereby preventing some vital function from unfolding. If the food we eat is rich in enzymes, vitamins, and minerals, it will add to our lives. If it is deficient in any of these elements, this will take away from the total life-force available to us. Vitamins, minerals, and hormones cannot work without the presence of enzymes.

Enzyme deficient diseases
The length and quality of life is directly proportional to the amount of available enzymes in the body. The level of amylase in human saliva is approximately 30 times more abundant in the average 25-year-old than the average 81-year-old. In contrast, whales and dolphins, who live in the perfectly balanced aquatic environment and live entirely on raw foods have no difference in cell enzyme composition in young and old (Murray MD, *Sea Energy Agriculture*).

If one were to analyze the bloodstreams of newborns and elderly persons, there would be little difference noted in the comparative blood levels of most vitamins and minerals in the infant and the old person. Amazingly, however, there are more than 100 times more enzymes present in the bloodstream of a newborn than that of an elderly person! This, to me, is an incredible, startling fact! Given this, can we then not look at premature old age, or for that matter, the aging process itself, as a biological condition with a major characteristic being pronounced enzyme deficiency?

Vibrant, healthy cells have high enzyme activity levels. Enzymes are the spark of life and are what makes living cells and tissues truly alive. It is a dubious strategy to expect energy and aliveness from life and then go about eating all that is dead and lifeless. Dr. Francis Pottenger's famous ten-year study showed just that. He fed one group of cats an enzyme-rich diet, and found these cats maintained their health and vigor throughout several generations. A second group of cats, who were fed a diet consisting of 80% cooked food for several generations. The group of cats, who were fed 80% cooked food, exhibited evidence of degenerative disease. Pottenger's data supported Howell's theories that raw food contains vital factors no longer present in cooked food. The SAD (Standard American Diet) has a much higher percentage of cooked and processed foods than most other diets, hence it does not come as a surprise to see that more than 70% of Americans are suffering from some form of degenerative disease. The excess intake of cooked fats leads to the exhaustion of the body's ability to manufacture sufficient amounts of lipase, the enzyme responsible for digesting fat. This in turn can lead to obesity, adult onset diabetes, and cardiovascular disease. Eskimos, on the other hand, can eat up to a pound of lipase-rich raw blubber each and every day and not have any signs or symptoms of cardiovascular disease. However, when Eskimos began to cook their fats like Westerners, they began to suffer from the degenerative diseases that the Western cultures do.

Another medical researcher, Dr. Paul Kauchakoff, MD, experimented with the effects of cooked and raw foods on the bloodstreams of humans. Dr. Kauchakoff found that eating cooked foods caused an immediate increase in the leucocyte (white blood) cell count in the bloodstream, whereas the same food eaten raw did not change blood physiology. Before this important experiment, medical dictum taught that this was a normal physiological event for leucocytes to increase in the blood and migrate to the intestines as soon as food entered the mouth. The strongest hypothesis formulated to explain this phenomenon is that in the body's wisdom, white blood cells collect enzymes from the body's enzyme reserves and migrate to the digestive system to aid in the digestion of the cooked food. Every cooked meal can then be seen as a significant stress on the immune system, speeding the exhaustion of enzymes and ultimately shortening your life.

Enzymeless diet speeds aging

Dr. James B Sumner, Nobel prize recipient and Professor of Biochemistry at Cornell University, wrote in his book *The Secret of Life-Enzymes*, that the "getting old feeling" after 40 is due to reduced enzyme levels throughout the body. Young cells contain 100 times more enzymes than the old cells. Old cells are filled with metabolic waste and toxins. In the textbook *Enzymes in Health and Disease*, co-edited by Dr. David Greenberg PhD, Chair of the Department of Biochemistry at the University of California School of Medicine at San Francisco, this editor suggests that for optimal health, longevity, and the reduction of many of the diseases of old age, the use of proteolytic (protein digesting) enzymes should begin about the age of 40 and should optimally continue for the rest of the life-span.

In a similar vein, Dr. Max Wolf, MD, in his book *Enzyme Therapy*, strongly endorses the use of plant-based enzymes. Dr. Wolf states: "Indigestion due to greasy foods is common… Plant-based enzymes are helpful for weak digestions common in old age, or for digestive disturbances. Enzymes are helpful with large rich meals or hard-to-digest foods. Preparations fortified with plant lipase, prevent postprandial (after eating) discomfort or gallbladder attacks."

Enzymes fight free radicals

Free radicals are not holdovers from the 1960s, but are highly-reactive, electrically-imbalanced molecules that damage other cells by trying to unite with them in a sort of sexual harassment on the cellular level. When this happens, the cell wall is ruptured and the contents of the cell spills out and begins a cascade of reactions that causes more free radicals to form. Free radical formation is not always pathological but is a natural event that occurs in the process of living. Eating poor foods and living an unhealthy lifestyle can increase free radical formation. However, our body manufactures special antioxidant enzymes (i.e., superoxide dismutase) to remove free radicals before they create cellular damage. In youth, our cells are able to produce sufficient amounts of the metabolic enzymes superoxide dismutase and catalase, which enable them to defend themselves by neutralizing free radicals. As we age we need to provide the cells with sufficient support, so that they can continue to maintain that balance.

Plant versus animal enzymes

Animal-based enzymes work very powerfully on food when the optimal acid-alkaline (pH) environment that these animal-based enzymes require is present. What animal enzyme manufacturers, and those that prescribe these products, do not tell you is that the optimal conditions necessary for animal-based enzymes to work optimally do not correspond to the actual *in vivo* (in the body) conditions of the human gastrointestinal tract. Outside of this narrow, optimal range, animal enzymes do not work as well as aspergillus plant-based enzymes.

Pepsin, which only digests protein, is taken from pig carcasses and works if (and only if) the acid environment stomach reaches a pH of 3 or less. This is not always the case, especially in humans who need supplemental pepsin in the first place. *Pancreatin*, which is taken from cow carcasses, works best in the neutral or slightly alkaline environment of the duodenum at a pH of between 7.8 and 8.3. These conditions are also not always present.

In contrast, plant-based aspergillus oryzae enzymes function well in the wide pH range actually found in the human gastrointestinal tract. Aspergillus oryzae plant enzymes are active in the stomach during the first 30 to 60 minutes of the meal. When the acidity of the lower (pyloric) stomach climbs, the aspergillus enzymes are temporarily inactivated. As it passes into the alkaline environment of the dueodenum, aspergillus becomes re-activated again.

Enzyme products help the "SAD" one

The National Digestive Diseases Information Clearinghouse in Bethesda, Maryland published these 1993 statistics for the US, as follows: 116,609 digestive system cancer deaths; 20 million cases of gallstones; 66 million reports of "heartburn" each month; 20 million cases of irritable bowel syndrome; 191,311 total deaths due to digestive disease;

22.3 million work-loss days due to chronic indigestion; 9 million work-loss days due to acute indigestion; 4.5 million hospitalizations due to indigestion; 13% of total hospitalizations due to digestive disorders; 5.8 million digestive system surgeries; and 7% of the total number of surgeries performed were digestive system related.

Indigestion brings in its malodorous trail a host of symptoms and discomforts such as heartburn, gas, bloatedness, nausea, burping, bad breath, body odors, headaches, abdominal pain, insomnia, nightmares, allergies, fatigue, constipation, diarrhea, irritable bowel syndrome, diverticulosis, cramps, spasms, skin problems, acne, pimples, food allergies, antacid dependency, post-meal mental fatigue, lack of concentration, memory loss, and nervousness. What are the harmful consequences of chronic indigestion? When food does not digest properly, starches go sour, proteins putrefy and fats turn rancid. Important nutrients become unavailable to the billions of cells that clamor for them. Excess acidity or alkalinity can set in, resulting in aches and pains and a loss of energy that is sometimes mistaken for psychological depression. The electro-voltage potential of your cells declines, leading to premature aging. To compensate for this generalized lack of energy some of us eat sugar or caffeine to "jump start" ourselves so we can "keep on going." If this negative cycle persists, we *will* keep on going—to an early grave.

Furthermore, chemical energy is stored in a molecule known as adenosine triphosphate (ATP). By way of enzymatic action, food is transformed into energy and then stored in the ATP molecules in our cells. The less efficient is our digestion, the less ATP energy will be created. Furthermore, when digestion is inefficient, fermenting and putrefying food has to be neutralized by our immune system, which requires ATP energy to do the cleansing.

The enzyme effect on allergies

Allergies are among the most common and costly of all health problems, afflicting an estimated 73 million people at a cost in excess of over 1.5 billion dollars a year. Nine percent of all patients seeking medical care at a physician's office do so for allergies. (*Asthma and other Allergic*

Disease, NIAID, NIH Publ. 79-387, 5/79) Allergies can be caused by an innumerable variety of substances, including food, pollen, dust, molds, drugs, cosmetics, toiletries, fabrics, poison ivy, etc. These allergens can enter your body through your food, the air, your skin, and even via medical injections.

Food allergies evoke a wide variety of symptoms, including fatigue, nervous tension, headaches, dizziness, nasal congestion, runny nose, itching, rashes, abdominal cramping, nausea, vomiting, and diarrhea. Foods high on the allergy list are milk, wheat, corn, eggs, seafood, and chocolate. Many people are also allergic to berries, citrus, and tomatoes. It is possible to be allergic to any food, including whole natural foods. However, I have observed that many people who are allergic to unsoaked or cooked seeds, nuts, and grains are no longer allergic to them when they are sprouted or soaked, or if they take food enzymes. Why does this positive change take place? The enzymes in these foods become enlivened with the sprouting process. The complex allergenic elements of these foods, i.e. the gluten found in wheat, become predigested and/or neutralized by the action of these enzymes.

Many foods contain these hard-to-digest elements. Dr. Howell cited experiments that showed that bacteria, yeast cells, large protein molecules, and fats can slip through the walls of the intestines and into the bloodstream. If this happens the already stressed immune system will not be able to deal with these undigested food elements and foreign proteins floating around. He further demonstrated that protective enzymes in the bloodstream break down these substances and absorb or neutralize them. In this connection, it was also found that if enzyme levels were too low, allergies developed. When supplemental enzymes were administered and the measured enzyme level in the blood had significantly increased, the allergies disappeared. The allergic reaction itself is the body's way to remove the allergen from the system. If this allergic reaction is suppressed by medication, then the body is forced to store the allergen in the body. The long-term effect of suppression is the eventual development of degenerative disease.

Dr. Cory Resnick, in *Plant Enzyme Therapy,* discusses practical approaches in treatment of food allergies: "By digesting dietary protein, plant enzymes administered orally at mealtime work to decrease the supply of antigenic macromolecules available to leak into the bloodstream. In addition, orally administered plant enzymes which have themselves been absorbed intact may help to 'digest' antigenic dietary proteins which they encounter in the bloodstream" (*Pizzome et al, '92*).

Enzyme fasting and healing
When you fast or go on a liquid diet of raw fruit and vegetable juices, your digestive system no longer has to produce enzymes. According to what Dr. Howell refers to as the "law of adaptive secretion," the enzyme potential, no longer directed into digesting food, can now be utilized by the general metabolic pool. These enzymes are now free to repair and rejuvenate the tissues and organs that need attention in other parts of the body. Many a seriously ill person has surprised family, friends, and doctors by healing themselves of seemingly incurable diseases when they adopted a total life-enhancing regime that included a high enzyme diet including supplementary enzymes, sufficient rest, appropriate exercise, positive mental attitude, and a conducive social and physical environment.

For a person who is run-down and toxic, it is not impossible to adopt such a program at home, but for those who are sick, the supervision of a competent health professional is strongly advised. One can also travel to the health centers that specialize in education and/or healing people who are dedicated to regaining their health. A few places in Europe include Josef Issel's Ringberg Clinic in West Germany, and Dr. Essen's Vita Nova in Sweden. In the Unites States, Hippocrates Health Institute of West Palm Beach, Florida provides a beautiful residential setting where one can learn by doing.

Can children use plant enzymes?
Most children have strong digestive systems. However, the fact that they can digest less-than-optimal cooked foods does not automatically make these foods ideal for the future unfolding of their maximum health

potential. Sure, kids will digest the foods served them and still be full of youthful energy, but the same health principles hold for children as they do for adults: namely, that the process of aging is accelerated when enzyme reserves are squandered by the burden of digesting excessive amounts of cooked food.

Plant enzymes and medication

If you are under medical care or taking oral medication of any kind, there are steps you should take to avoid any inactivation of an enzyme supplement by your medication. Sprinkle plant enzyme powder *on the food itself* instead of taking the capsules or powder directly into your body. Make sure, however, that the food has cooled down a bit or else the enzyme powder will be damaged by the high heat of your food. In this way, the predigestive action of the enzymes will work directly on the food and not have to come in contact with the drugs that may be in your stomach.

Despite the long-overdue surfacing of the truth about enzymes, don't be surprised if your family doctor still downplays the importance or even the existence of enzymes in foods. Traditionally, segments of the medical community take a conservative posture on many issues. In fact, the majority of doctors, dieticians and nutritionists do not fully appreciate the contribution of food enzymes to health maintenance and the prevention of disease. At the conclusion of this chapter you will probably know more about food enzymes than most physicians!

Do plant enzymes survive gut acids?

Less than one fifth of all medical schools in the United States teach even the elementary aspects of nutrition. Of those that do teach it, the true role of food enzymes is rarely if ever taught. According to the prevailing accepted dictum, enzymes found in foods are destroyed by the hydrochloric acid of the stomach and are virtually no use in the digestive economy. However, Dr. Howell has shown that as soon as particular food is masticated in the mouth, the enzymes begin to digest the food. This has been confirmed by Finnish Nobel Prize winner Artturi

Virtanen. When the food reaches the first part of the stomach, (upper cardiac stomach) the food enzymes are still actively working. It takes up to 50 minutes for the hydrochloric acid level to rise to the critical level where the acidity of the hydrochloric acid could inactivate the food enzymes in the food. Until this level is reached, the food enzymes are still working. What is more, not all foods stimulate hydrochloric acid production appreciably. Foods like fruit, spouts, grasses and many raw vegetables do not cause hydrochloric acid production to increase rapidly or in any great quantity. In this environment enzymes present in food have a longer time to do their work. According to Howell, even though saliva enzymes shut off in the presence of acid, food enzymes are not markedly disturbed.

After taking enzyme supplements, many people immediately feel a difference in the ease in which their food is digested. They also report an overall boost in their energy level. Others do not report any dramatic subjective improvement. The latter case is probably due to the relatively good health enjoyed already or the fact that the "blood of youth" has not as yet faded. Whether you feel any immediate subjective improvements in your health as a result of taking enzymes is not as important as your understanding how enzymes do their work of enhancing digestion and assimilation, boosting the immune system and contributing to your body's total vitality.

In conclusion

Our longevity and our well-being could be increased if we ate more whole foods with an emphasis on uncooked foods.

Dr. Howell's powerful words say it all:

"There is no other mechanism in the body except enzyme action to protect the body from any hazard. It is ambiguous to say that "nature cures" when we must know that the only machinery in the body to do anything is enzyme action. Hormones do not work. Vitamins cannot do any work. Minerals were not made to do any work. Proteins cannot work. Nature does not work. Only enzymes are made for work."

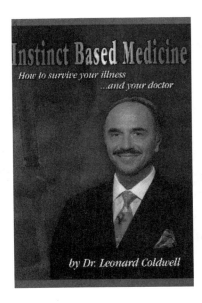

Instinct Based Medicine™

Dr. Leonard Coldwell is a health researcher who has spent his career addressing the root cause of disease/illness and how to help patients get rid of the cause of the illness. He discovered that the only way to help his patients was to help them to help themselves, which led him to be known as the "health coach." He does not care about the symptoms of disease/illness because he only addresses the root cause of the illness.

—**Dr. Coldwell** is my personal physician in Europe and his input over the years was extremely valuable for me and the creation of my mega best selling book, *Natural Cures They Don't Want You to Know About.* Dr. Leonard Coldwell is the original natural cures doctor. We are in constant contact, consulting with each other all the time. I am glad that Dr. Leonard Coldwell is now willing to share with the world his secrets for health and healing. In *Instinct Based Medicine*, Dr. Coldwell uncovers the horrifying truth about the medical profession and shows us how to find and eliminate the life circumstances, behaviors, decisions and actions we live with on a daily basis that endanger our health.

This ground breaking book will reach and help millions of people! I ask you to support Dr. Coldwell in his approach to educating and protecting the public from the dangers of modern medicine to give everyone the tools to control their own life and health. Please support this book and help spread the message. I wish my dear friend, Dr. Leonard Coldwell, the biggest success with his book *Instinct Based Medicine*!
—Kevin Trudeau
NY Times Best Selling Author and Consumer advocate May 2008

Dr. Leonard's book may be purchased at
http://www.instinctbasedmedicine.com/